The Forensic Examination and Interpretation of Tool Marks

The Forensic Examination and Interpretation of Tool Marks

David Baldwin
Baldwin Forensic Consultancy, Formerly of Forensic Science Service Ltd, London

John Birkett
Formerly of Forensic Science Service Ltd, London

Owen Facey
Staffordshire University

Gilleon Rabey
Formerly of Forensic Science Service Ltd, London

WILEY Blackwell

This edition first published 2013 © 2013 by John Wiley & Sons, Ltd

Registered office: John Wiley & Sons, Ltd, The Atrium, Southern Gate, Chichester, West Sussex, PO19 8SQ, UK

Editorial offices: 9600 Garsington Road, Oxford, OX4 2DQ, UK

The Atrium, Southern Gate, Chichester, West Sussex, PO19 8SQ, UK

111 River Street, Hoboken, NJ 07030-5774, USA

For details of our global editorial offices, for customer services and for information about how to apply for permission to reuse the copyright material in this book please see our website at www.wiley.com/wiley-blackwell.

The right of the authors to be identified as the authors of this work has been asserted in accordance with the UK Copyright, Designs and Patents Act 1988.

Library of Congress Cataloging-in-Publication Data

Baldwin, David, Forensic consultant.

  The forensic examination and interpretation of tool marks / David Baldwin, John Birkett, Owen Facey, Gilleon Rabey.

       pages cm

  Includes bibliographical references and index.

  ISBN 978-1-119-97246-4 (cloth) – ISBN 978-1-119-97245-7 (pbk.) 1. Tools–Identification.
2. Evidence, Criminal. 3. Forensic sciences. 4. Criminal investigation.   I. Title.

  HV8077.5.T66B35 2013

  363.25′62–dc23

                                                                        2012050081

A catalogue record for this book is available from the British Library.

Wiley also publishes its books in a variety of electronic formats. Some content that appears in print may not be available in electronic books.

Cover image: Left: iStockphoto / Pixel_Pig; Right: iStockphoto / Viktor Pryymachuk; Bottom: author supply

Set in 10.5/13pt Times by Laserwords Private Limited, Chennai, India

First Impression 2013

Contents

About the Authors

David Baldwin

David joined the Metropolitan Police Forensic Science Laboratory (MPFSL) in London in 1974 and worked in the General Chemistry and Blood Alcohol Departments. In 1977 he gained a BSc (Honours) degree in Chemistry from the Polytechnic of North London. In 1996 the MPFSL was merged with the Home Office Forensic Science Service (FSS), with that organisation ultimately becoming The Forensic Science Service®, where David worked until its closure in March 2012. He was the Principal Scientist for Marks in The Forensic Science Service, having been a Senior Court Reporting Scientist for many years involved in the examination of cases involving manufacturing marks, including those on plastic film items, tool and footwear marks, paint and glass. In the role of Principal Scientist he was responsible to senior management for quality and technical aspects of marks' work in the organisation. Between 2005 and 2012 David served as the Chair of the steering committee of the European Network of Forensic Science Institutes (ENFSI) Working Group Marks, helping to standardise and improve forensic science examinations throughout Europe.

John Birkett

Like David, John started work at the MPFSL in 1974, after gaining a BSc (Honours) degree in Chemistry from Birmingham University. He worked in the Drug Section for a short time before transferring to the then General Chemistry Department, which was eventually to become known as 'Marks and Traces'. Here he was involved in the examination of cases involving contact traces such as paint and glass as well as footwear marks, locks and keys and, of course, tool marks until the FSS closed in March 2012. As a Senior Court Reporting Scientist, he worked on many thousands of cases involving tool marks for police forces throughout England and Wales as well as checking the work and findings of his colleagues in many more. John has given expert testimony in many courts from Magistrates' to Coroners', including the Central Criminal Court (also known as The Old Bailey). In the late 1970s the MPFSL set up a database of tool marks from unsolved offences to look for otherwise unsuspected links between scenes of crime. The marks were also screened against tools submitted from offenders. This became part of the Marks' Intelligence Index database and John was responsible for running that until 2011. Between 1995 and 2003 John served on the steering committee of the ENFSI Working Group Marks.

Owen Facey

Owen graduated from London University in 1964 with a PhD in Physical Chemistry, having already obtained a BSc (Honours) degree in Chemistry, and spent the next five years as a research fellow in what are now called 'condensed matter materials' in England, Canada and the United States. On returning to the United Kingdom he joined the Metropolitan Police Forensic Science Laboratory in 1970 and worked in the General Chemistry Department, which undertook the developing areas of footwear and tool marks as well as chemical analysis of all materials other than drugs and poisons. Tool marks became one of Owen's main interests, although he also reported chemical traces, footwear marks and manufacturing marks, including those on plastic bags. Owen was a Senior Court Reporting Scientist responsible for managing a team and carried out some research and development work. He was also involved in writing the procedures used in the initial accreditation of various departments such as chemistry, documents, firearms, traffic accidents and metallurgy. He left the Laboratory in 1999, which had become the Forensic Science Service in 1996. Owen became a consultant forensic scientist working mainly for Forensic Alliance, now LGC Forensics, and Forensic Access. In this period he undertook defence as well as prosecution work, retiring from active casework in 2010; since 2007 he has been a research fellow at Staffordshire University.

Gilleon Rabey

Gilleon started work at the London Laboratory of the Forensic Science Service in March 1998 with a first class BSc (Honours) in Human Biology, which she gained in 1997 from the University of Leeds. Her first job was as a DNA Analyst, working in the busy DNA Casework Unit, processing DNA samples from serious and high profile crimes. She progressed to reporting National DNA Database matches and a future as a forensic biologist beckoned. The unusual move to reporting tool and footwear marks occurred following the successful completion of her MSc degree in Forensic Archaeological Science in 2002 from University College London, where she developed an interest in tool marks (in bones). She became a Senior Court Reporting Scientist, also specialising in lock and key comparisons, and was involved in writing support manuals and standard operating procedures for tool mark examiners prior to leaving the FSS at the end of 2011, preceding its closure in 2012.

Series Foreword

Essentials of Forensic Science

The world of forensic science is changing at a very fast pace in terms of the provision of forensic science services, the development of technologies and knowledge and the interpretation of analytical and other data as it is applied within forensic practice. Practicing forensic scientists are constantly striving to deliver the very best for the judicial process and as such need a reliable and robust knowledge base within their diverse disciplines. It is hoped that this book series will provide a resource by which such knowledge can be underpinned for both students and practitioners of forensic science alike.

It is the objective of this book series to provide a valuable resource for forensic science practitioners, educators and others in that regard. The books developed and published within this series come from some of the leading researchers and practitioners in their fields and will provide essential and relevant information to the reader.

Niamh Nic Daéid
Series Editor

Foreword

I had the great pleasure to collaborate with the authors when I joined the now defunct Forensic Science Service (FSS) in 2000. I was hired to carry out research and to work with forensic practitioners on interpretation issues. DNA evidence was at the forefront of all minds, but my forensic background and practice was with marks. The authors of this book, colleagues from the marks' and traces' department of the FSS, gave me forensic asylum and allowed me to act at times as their 'interpretation troublemaker'. It led us to confront (often foolish) ideas and to develop compromises that we have tried to promote within the profession at large.

Four words are used in the Introduction to describe the expected qualities of a forensic statement: logical, transparent, balanced and robust. They also apply to this book, and allow the field to move from a set of whispered secrets within the trade to a structured body of knowledge from which one can be trained to be an examiner. In a long-awaited addition to any good forensic library, the authors contribute, in a very accessible form, their extensive knowledge and experience in this specialized area. Unfortunately, and for decades, the field of tool marks' examination has not received specific attention. It is viewed by many that treatment by pure analogy to the consideration of footwear marks or marks left by firearms on bullets or cartridge cases is sufficient when dealing with the other tools. The analogy carries merit up to a certain point, but this book very elegantly shows its limits and invites the reader to realise that this area of forensic science is a discipline on its own.

Tool marks were fully recognized by the early pioneers of forensic science as the main means of reconstructing events and helping establish indirect relationships with potential culprits (typically through the size of tools). Alphonse Bertillon is probably the first to have published a full detailed case study of the tool marks recovered from the desk of a murdered financier (*Archives d'Anthropologie crimininelle et de Médecine légale*, 1909, 753–782). Rodolphe-Archibald Reiss, in his 1911 book *Manuel de police scientifique I. Vols et homicides*, makes extensive reference to their contribution in investigations and presents documented examples from his practice on offences against property. One of the first murder investigations by Reiss, in 1911, dealt with striated marks left by a hatchet on the skull of the victim, a Mrs Seewer. Compared with any other marks that can be left by a perpetrator on a scene, none speaks more about the offence itself than potential recovered tool marks.

This book's Introduction provides some definitions used within the area and elements of good training and practice that are developed in subsequent chapters. In Chapter 2, the reader is then taken through the manufacturing process of tools. This is a key component that is often minimized or ignored in training. To become a proficient examiner, there is a requirement to learn about this topic by, for example, visiting manufacturing sites and not working from an assumption that 'it has probably been manufactured that way'.

Chapter 3 conveys an essential message to all investigating agencies: detailed knowledge of the types of marks that can be obtained from crime scenes is paramount to success. Covering levering, gripping, cutting, impact or saw marks (with or without striations) both on objects and on body parts, the chapter deals with all types of criminal activities that lead to tool marks and the operational constraints to secure them properly. It will convince any forensic scientist of the appealing diversity of the work of a tool mark examiner. Chapter 4 deals with the planning and initial examination.

The entire volume is full of operational advice and good practices that will speak to all practitioners. It also invites them to carry out a pre-assessment of the case in close collaboration with the submitting agency and forensic scientists from other disciplines e.g. drugs, traces (paint, fibres, . . .), biological traces (blood, saliva, epithelial cells, . . .), fingerprints. In today's forensic science where the risks of contextual bias are used as a reason to separate the laboratory from the field definitively, this chapter delivers a crucial message: a close connection between the submitting agency and examiners is the only way to provide a value-added service from a multidisciplinary perspective.

The potential contribution of this field is made perfectly clear: (1) in an evaluative mode—to help associate recovered marks with potential tools and (2) the often neglected investigative contribution—offering leads in the investigation as to the type and size of the tool(s) involved and as an intelligence instrument (through scene linking). The detailed laboratory examination of tool marks is then covered in Chapter 5. Again, this chapter gives very astute practical advice that has not been disclosed elsewhere to my knowledge.

Chapter 6 deals with the interpretation and evaluation of the findings. The authors give their opinions as to the best practice. It is suggested that a two-stage approach is adopted: firstly, an interpretation decision is made as to whether or not the compared marks can be deemed to be *matching* or *not matching*; secondly, the practitioner will assign—or evaluate—the weight to be assigned to the 'matching' cases (the 'not matching' ones leading to a conclusion of exclusion). The difficulties associated with the evaluation are clearly exposed and serve as an excellent basis for adopting a logical approach. However, I would not say that I adhere to all the proposals made by the authors, as I need to maintain my 'troublemaker' status. For example, it is my contention that reporting conclusive links in an absolute way should stop rather than continue on, if we want to confer a scientific status to the discipline. All forensic evidence should be considered as corroborative, even physical fits. Also, I would ban completely terms such as *random*, *individual*, or *unique* from the vocabulary of any forensic examiner. Finally, I would link the steps of the reporting scales strictly to declared ranges of likelihood ratios. In this chapter, the authors make their point in such an open and transparent manner that it creates a healthy room for debate.

Chapter 7 focuses on manufacturing marks (with an obvious focus on tool marks) with a few case studies. The reader will appreciate the range of cases, marks and associated specialized knowledge this discipline covers. Various types of physical fits are dealt with in Chapter 8, with the correct emphasis again on the importance of the scene of crime examination. Plastic film examination (Chapter 9) can help in cases involving wrapping and packaging. Not only could the questions relate to the source, but also to events of a reconstruction and the use of the material, whether it is pigmented or transparent plastic bags, wrapping film or self-adhesive tapes. This chapter brings home one key message that is applicable to the entire book: a detailed knowledge of the manufacturing chain is required in order assess properly the potential contribution of such examinations and to interpret the forensic findings observed.

This book provides a short but detailed overview of the specialized subject of tool marks' examination. It cuts to the chase and conveys with passion the key foundations of the discipline. It is written by four very enthusiastic and experienced practitioners, who master the provision of evidence from crime scene to courtroom. They agreed to share their vast knowledge acquired though their dozens of years spent as colleagues and friends on specialized casework. They bring to the field an essential and collegial building block. Not only are the technical aspects thoroughly covered, with a lot of practical advice, but also, and on an equal footing, the authors put to the forefront the questions of scene examination, establishment of the exact requirements, pre-assessment and case assessment and interpretation. This book is aimed at students in forensic science, but, without any doubt, will become a standard textbook for all forensic scientists dealing with tool marks.

Christophe Champod
University of Lausanne
School of Criminal Justice, Institute of Forensic Science

Preface

Much has been published in the way of scientific papers on tool marks, but there has been very little written in the way of a definitive text on the matter, unlike footwear or tyre marks, which have several books dedicated to each topic. With a collective 129 years of experience of working in forensic science in the United Kingdom, and having examined many thousands of tool marks between us, it seemed logical for us to write a book on the subject. This book is written as part of a series for forensic science students and aims to summarise the benefit of our experience, detailing what we feel is best practice, based on established and validated methods used in the United Kingdom. Reference will be made to the practices of other countries, but the methodology may vary, not least because of what is acceptable by the jurisdiction of the courts. We hope that this book will not only capture the interest of potential future tool mark examiners, but also raise the awareness of those involved in associated professions, such as investigators or barristers, who may never have encountered tool marks before.

Tool marks offer the potential for obtaining very good evidence. They can be left at any crime scene, in any substrate, where an offender has used a tool to commit an offence. Almost by definition, tool marks must be crime marks, as people tend not to jemmy their own doors open! Nor are they likely to happen by accidental contact, as some force is normally involved in their production. Tool marks can offer information about the size and type of the tool responsible and have the potential to contain gross and microscopic detail that has been produced by irregularities on the surface of the tool responsible. The irregularities on the surface of a tool relate to features of their manufacture and use. Any features visible in a mark can be used to exclude or show a level of association with a particular tool recovered during a criminal investigation.

The field of tool marks does not stop at the comparison of conventional burgling tools with marks recovered from scenes of crime. If something has been hit, punctured or cut with a tool, there is potential for marks to be left that could, theoretically, be compared. Anyone who has watched archaeological programmes will have seen bones being examined for marks made by butchery or flint arrowheads and swords, or wooden structures having marks left by 'axes'. In tool marks, almost anything is possible as the authors have encountered much variety in the types of tool used and substrates marks have been made in.

Contact with police officers and scene examiners over the years has shown that many do not appreciate the evidential value of tool marks (potentially the equivalent of a 'full ident' in fingerprint terms) or what can be achieved by retrieving and examining them properly under laboratory conditions. Sadly, all too many tool marks are left *in situ* at the crime scene, after a presumption has been made that they are too poor quality to contain any detail, based on, for example, size, depth or substrate, without examining them microscopically to confirm that this is or is not the case.

It is hoped that in this book we can highlight how small an area the experienced tool mark examiner can work their 'miracles' on, if there is detail in a mark that can be visualised and the correct tool has been recovered. The perception can be that a tool mark needs to show the full width and be deeply impressed, but that is only a small proportion of viable marks that may be found at a scene. Shallow, partial impressed marks can be just as useful, if found and recovered. In addition, cut marks, grazing marks and sliding/slippage marks should not be ignored, even though they do not obviously show the shape or size of the tool responsible. If it can be recovered a mark can be examined to determine what made it and to compare with marks from other scenes or tools from suspects. There are no guarantees, but without a detailed examination in the laboratory, it would be all too possible to dismiss the marks as unsuitable.

In addition to the quality of detail that a tool mark may contain (so long as it is located and recovered from the crime scene in the first place), there are some other very important factors that must be considered in order to obtain the right results and the strongest level of evidence possible, which we will cover in more detail in the book. First and foremost, any casting materials used by scene or tool mark examiners need to be able to replicate fine detail in a mark. Proper lighting and having the best equipment available are also essential to resolve and enhance the detail.

However, all this would still be fruitless in the absence of a fully competent tool mark practitioner who knows how to use the equipment properly to obtain the best results. The examiner has to be able to visualise marks on a whole range of materials and to get them into a form suitable for presenting to a comparison microscope (comparator). To carry out the comparison it is also necessary to determine how the marks were made to know which part of the tool could have been responsible and to make suitable test marks.

In order to interpret the results of any comparisons, the examiner should know how tools are made and the type of detail that can be produced by different manufacturing processes, as well as the type of detail that can be acquired through wear and damage as the tool is used.

In some countries, tool mark examination falls within the purview of firearm examiners, since the comparison of striations on fired bullets and firing pin marks on cartridge cases are also tool mark examinations, albeit specialised ones. In other countries, examiners within departments of 'general chemistry', 'criminalistics' or 'marks and traces' deal with tool marks. Whichever department in a laboratory deals with tool marks is not important so long as the examiners are fully trained and competent, and maintain and update their knowledge and competence regularly. There is a need for the examiners to deal with more than just the odd case now and then and concentrating the examinations to a relatively small group has its benefits. Since 1995, the ENSI Marks' Working Group has enabled information to be exchanged by means of regular bulletins and conferences that are open to examiners from all over the world.

Although not traditional 'tool' marks as described above, we have included physical fit and manufacturing mark examinations in the book (including those involving plastic films such as bags and tapes) as there are certain aspects of tool mark examination that apply to them as well. Either knowledge of detail left by the machinery during manufacture is required to evaluate any findings or tool mark techniques are employed to carry out a comparison. These are other areas of forensic examination that are not commonly encountered in scientific text and so it was felt necessary to include them for completeness.

We are grateful to the input we have had throughout our careers from colleagues in the Metropolitan Police Forensic Science Laboratory (MPFSL) and the Forensic Science Service (FSS) and from laboratories in other countries, particularly in Europe, who have added to our knowledge. Also, thanks should be given to various firms who, over the years, have allowed access to their factories to see tools being made. We thank our former colleagues from the Forensic Science Service, Denise Kelly for checking draft material for relevance and accuracy and Dr Philip Davis for allowing us to use photographs taken on a factory visit. In addition, we must not forget our spouses, Deborah Baldwin, Carol Birkett, Kikuko Facey and Liam Rabey, family and friends for their support, especially in the hectic two months or so as the book finally came together. Gilleon would particularly like to thank her mother Nicola Moulds and other obliging babysitters (Katie Dalziel, Paula Keay, Alistair and Andrew Moulds), for looking after her son Malcolm so that she could work on the book without interruption. She would also like to thank Chris Hadkiss, who was DNA Unit Manager at the Forensic Science

Service in 2002, for giving her the opportunity to move to the Marks' and Traces' Department. John would also like to thank his mother-in-law for allowing him to mock up a burglary in action on her windows and doors and to his wife Carol for photographing him in action!

David Baldwin
John Birkett
Owen Facey
Gilleon Rabey

About the Companion Website

This book is accompanied by a companion website:

www.wiley.com/go/baldwin/forensictoolmarks

The website includes:

- Powerpoints of all figures from the book for downloading
- PDFs of tables from the book

1

Introduction

1.1 Overview of contents

The term 'tool mark examination' is often applied to cover a wide range of possible forensic examinations. However, whilst the term implies that you must have some type of tool or instrument before you can proceed, this is not the case at all as we shall see. Throughout the book we will use the term 'tool' to cover all instruments, tools or other objects that have come into contact with another surface.

As the term suggests, it primarily applies to examinations involving marks that have been made by a tool or tools used by a person in order to commit an offence, where usually both the scene mark(s) and suspect tool(s) are available to the examiner for consideration, to determine whether or not the tool submitted was the one used. Chapters 2–6 will mainly deal with this type of typical tool mark examination, concentrating on the important aspects used by the examiner such as how tools are made and what features may be found on their surfaces, the type of tool marks that can be found at scenes of crime, the laboratory techniques that can be used to examine them and how results can be interpreted and evaluated. The principles that we will cover in these chapters, as well as here in Chapter 1, also provide a solid framework for the scientific investigation of other related forensic examinations described.

The basis of all tool mark examinations is that when one object comes into contact with a softer material, then evidence of the contact may result. Put simply, if the contact forces the two objects together without any movement then an impressed mark in the softer material will result; this may be a direct representation of the surface of the harder object that has been in contact. If however, there is some form of movement between the two objects then a dynamic mark will result. The dynamic mark will consist of a series of parallel

The Forensic Examination and Interpretation of Tool Marks, First Edition.
David Baldwin, John Birkett, Owen Facey and Gilleon Rabey.
© 2013 John Wiley & Sons, Ltd. Published 2013 by John Wiley & Sons, Ltd.

lines, which are often referred to as striations (made up of 'striae'). In general terms there are four main types of action that produce striated marks:

- sliding marks, which are sometimes also known as scratch marks, for example where a tool slips across the surface;

- cutting marks, where a single bladed tool such as a knife slices through an object;

- cutting marks, where a double bladed tool is used to sever an object;

- stabbing marks, where a tool is forced into a material.

In many instances a mark will consist of a combination of both impressed and dynamic detail, both of which have been produced by and directly relate to surface features on the harder object at the time the mark was made.

'Tool marks' therefore could also be found on the surface of a variety of manufactured items. This includes marks on the surface of those very tools and instruments that have been used to commit an offence. Hand tools such as screwdrivers, case openers and bolt cutters, to name but a few, are mass produced items that are shaped, moulded and finished by various processes during manufacturing. The machines, moulds and other equipment that form a finished hand tool are 'tools' themselves (albeit larger ones) and have the ability to leave marks of various descriptions on the finished manufactured item. Assessing how these manufacturing marks on the surface of tools were made and their evidential significance is a fundamental stage in the interpretation and evaluation of routine tool mark comparisons.

Therefore, it follows that other mass produced items will also have 'tool marks' upon their surfaces. For example, items such as screws, nuts and nails, where the item has been somehow shaped, moulded, gripped or cut to achieve the final shape and finish. However, for the purposes of this book, these will be referred to as 'manufacturing marks' and when considered alongside typical tool marks, the more general term 'marks' will be used. (This should not be confused with other forensic disciplines where marks are examined such as fingerprints, footwear marks or tyre marks.) In a forensic examination, such manufactured items may be seized from a crime scene and there is a necessity to compare them with a suspect population of similar items. In these sorts of circumstances, the tool mark detail on the surfaces of the items under examination needs to be assessed, and an evaluation made on whether or not they have come from the same source. For examinations such as these, the same equipment and techniques used for routine tool mark examination can be applied. The main difference is in how the results are interpreted and evaluated, which will be discussed in Chapter 7, although the same fundamental principles that we will see in Chapter 6 still apply.

In this book we will also cover what are known as 'physical fits'. This term refers to broken or torn items where the pieces can be demonstrated to have once been joined together, and therefore formed part of the same item. What the item is and how it was broken/torn can alter the information and laboratory techniques used in order to reach a conclusion. In general though, physical fit examinations fall into four main categories.

1. Broken items that can be obviously fitted back together; otherwise known as 'jigsaw' fits. A tool mark examiner would not necessarily be required to demonstrate this sort of physical fit.

2. Broken items where the pieces require routine tool mark examination techniques to demonstrate that the pieces fit together and thus to form a conclusion. The detail may require a microscopic comparison and use of casting.

3. Broken, torn or cut items where knowledge of manufacture and type of marks left on the surface of the item need to be taken into account in order to support a fit. Typically, these sorts of examinations require techniques more commonly associated with routine tool mark examinations or manufacturing marks, particularly those relating to plastic film items.

4. Items that were originally fitted together or were in contact for a period of time. Typically these examinations involve a consideration of what material has been transferred or is a result of the contact.

The categories of physical fit that fall under the auspices of tool mark or manufacturing mark examinations will be dealt with in Chapter 8.

Plastic manufactured items, such as plastic film, bags and adhesive tape, can also exhibit features of manufacture caused by the machinery and processes used to make them. As with other mass-produced items such as screws, examinations tend to focus on whether crime scene and suspect items came from the same source. However, in this particular area, different examination techniques are normally applied in order to visualise the detail (but the need to understand how the detail has originated during the manufacturing process remains the same). Another critical factor in the interpretation and evaluation of these sorts of manufacturing marks is knowledge of how rapidly the detail changes. Chapter 9 will cover aspects of forensic examination in relation to the manufacture of plastic film items, including physical fits (as described above under category three) involving this sort of material.

Whilst this book aims to cover a wide range of examination types encountered in this particular field of forensic science, it cannot be a catch all for all of the weird, wonderful and unusual examinations that the authors have encountered in their collective 129 years of forensic experience. However, the fundamental principles of more typical marks' examinations, which we shall describe in this book, can be applied to any type of examination that falls, no matter how tenuously, into the categories of marks described. Our aim is to cover a broad selection of more commonly encountered examination types and some tried and tested, best practice techniques and methods based on our knowledge and experience of doing work of this kind. However, such work is not without its limitations and Chapter 10 will attempt to capture some of the ways in which other experts in this field are striving to make improvements.

1.2   A brief history of tool marks

At this juncture, it is useful to put tool mark examination into an historical context, as it is a traditional area of work that has been in use for longer than may be expected. There has been an appreciation that marks can be related back to tools from early times, although there were few written texts on the subject. One frequently quoted example comes from 12th century China, where the different shapes of wound caused by cutting instruments such as sickles were considered but it had little impact on the courts, even in China. The first book to have a major effect was written by Hans Gross in 1891, published in 1893 as two volumes, entitled *Handbuch für Untersuchungsrichter als System der Kriminalistik*. This was later translated into various languages, including English (see Gross, 1907) and has been republished many times.

Gross was a professor of law at the University of Graz in Austria and was also a practising judge. The book was written from his experience as a judge and details some of the best physical, as distinct from circumstantial, evidence that was presented. Tool marks are not given in a specific chapter but feature under the heading of *Theft – Burglary and House Breaking*, in Chapter 17. In this Gross says that it is necessary to describe, record (here by drawing) and take mouldings of all the damage done by the thief. The example is given of a tool, where the impressed tip detail indicated that a screwdriver, rather than a chisel, had been used and examination with a hand lens showed that one corner was damaged. A sketch was made and later a screwdriver used in another burglary was connected to this scene using the recorded information. There is no mention of using microscopes here but they are mentioned in Chapter 5 Section vii, dealing with firearms together with a comparison microscope. This goes with the caution that '...microscopic examinations can only be made by really skilled experts'.

All the basic steps of tool mark examination are present in this work and it remained in print until 1934. During the period 1891–1934, the courts increasingly recognised the value of scientific evidence but there were no large laboratories in existence and equipment was both limited and often awkward to use. After 1945 there was a large surge in scientific research, both in universities and industry. Forensic science benefited from this and the investigation of tool marks and firearms was improved through the development of better designed equipment, especially optical equipment.

In 1953 Paul L. Kirk, who was by that time a Professor at the University of California in forensic science, wrote an influential textbook called *Crime Investigation*, which includes sections on tool mark examination. He recognised the need to cast marks found at scenes of crime, when the item with the mark cannot be taken to a laboratory and suggested ways of achieving this. By the time of the last update and reprint in 1974, two-pack silicone materials were being suggested for casting, with the added comment that there was the need to colour the surface to obtain good reflectivity for comparison purposes. There are detailed discussions relating to types of tools and the importance of what are now called class characteristics together with individual characteristic detail.

The book makes a clear distinction between 'compression marks', called impressed marks in this book, and 'sliding marks', here called dynamic or striated marks or further divided into sliding, cutting or stab marks depending on the action used. The method given for the examination of impressed marks is to use macro photography of the individual scene mark and the test mark, then to use side by side comparison of the photographic images. A comparison microscope (also known as a comparator or comparison macroscope[1]) with long focal length lenses is suggested for examining striated marks, with the comment that photography using the comparator is not always successful. Examination of physical fits is also included in the text.

There is a discussion of what is meant by a 'tool mark match', together with an increasing set of references to papers dealing with this topic in the reprints. There is recognition of the problems involved in 'matching' and the need for training and experience. In relation to striated marks, although by implication impressed marks as well, Kirk says 'There is a need for conservatism – no witness can truthfully state "This is the only tool on earth that could have made this mark"'. In the 1974 edition there is a reference to the work by Biasotti (1964), *The Principles of Evidence Evaluation as Applied to Firearms and Tool Mark Identification*, which contains some of the first references for objective methods for evaluating striated marks.

In 1958 J.E. Davis published *An Introduction to Toolmarks, Firearms and the Striagraph*. This gave more information than Kirk's book but, apart from introducing the striagraph, which did not enter general use, added little new.

---

[1] The term 'comparator' will be the one mainly used throughout this book.

While Kirk makes clear in his introduction that his book was written for 'laboratory criminalists', most of the later authors write for more general audiences. H.J. Walls, a director of the Metropolitan Police Forensic Science Laboratory, London, UK, wrote a book entitled *Forensic Science: An Introduction to Scientific Crime Detection*, the first edition appearing in 1968. He states in the introduction that the book is intended for non-specialists. There is a general discussion of tool marks, which does not go into any great detail about the methods used in their examination. In dealing with the problem of matching marks, he noted that there is rarely a 'perfect' match between test and questioned marks. In an unreferenced aside on striated marks he notes that tests in the United States showed that a correspondence of over 70% of the striae could be found for suitable marks made by the same tool but was less than 25% in marks made by different tools.

In 1969 the Association of Firearms and Tool Mark Examiners (AFTE) was formed in the United States. This provided a forum for those examiners, separate from the various forensic science groups already in existence. Its journal and publications did much to raise the profile of this area of forensic work and, eventually, to promote an international approach.

Since that time, forensic science has expanded as a university subject and a number of textbooks have been written to meet the demands of these courses. They often seek to be informative for other groups as well, such as scene of crime examiners, police and the legal profession, but rarely go into much detail about tool mark examination. Given the problems associated with interpreting and evaluating tool mark evidence this is, perhaps, not that surprising. A different reason lies in the developments in analysing body fluids and materials, where it is now possible to discriminate between millions of people in the best circumstances. At a crime scene these biological materials would be sought first, as they have a tendency to degrade and decompose and so could be rapidly lost, depending on the circumstances of the case and environmental conditions. This type of evidence can also often provide significant answers to an investigation rapidly. Generally tool mark evidence will not degrade and so collecting it may not be considered a priority. In some instances though, it may not be collected at all, which may be because it has not been detected or because a conscious decision has been made.

Preconceived ideas about limitations in the value or usefulness of tool mark evidence, along with the time and cost associated in examining it, may all be factors in its demise as a key forensic discipline, at least currently in the United Kingdom. However, tool marks can often provide vital and strong evidence of association as well as eliminate a suspect item, which can prove critical as an investigation progresses. What we think has been lacking, and which we will seek to provide in this book, is a text that deals predominantly with tool mark examination as it is presently practised, to help raise general awareness of the capabilities of this type of evidence.

1.3   General aspects of marks' comparison

At a fundamental level, a marks' comparison can be considered to be a comparison of the 'unknown' with the 'known'. The unknown items are those bearing marks recovered from the crime scene, which could be casts or original items. The known is a control item, which could be one taken from the suspect, such as a tool, or a population of items for reference, such as a bag of screws or roll of plastic bags that has been recovered during the course of an investigation for comparison.

The aim of the comparison process is therefore to determine what features and detail of the crime scene mark(s) differ or correspond to those on the control item(s). However, it is a fairly straightforward process to do a comparison of features, but much more difficult to interpret what the outcome means if one does not know what the features and detail are or how they were obtained. One of the most important aspects of any marks' examination is having equipment and techniques that allow you to visualise the, often microscopic, detail so that you are best placed to evaluate the significance of the findings.

Another critical aspect of a comparison is to understand the manufacturing processes associated with the 'control' item. There are three classes of features that an examiner will need to consider.

Class features	Features that are common to all items of a particular type.
Sub-class features	Features that are not unique to one particular item, but allow some discrimination between groups of tools with the same class features. They arise during manufacture, but are not necessarily introduced deliberately. The source of sub-class features may change over time.
Individual/unique	Characteristic features arising at random during the manufacturing process or through normal use.

To interpret and evaluate the findings it is therefore necessary to know and understand the types of features and detail produced during manufacture and use, how they will be represented in a mark and how to differentiate between the different types, as this will determine what you are able to say about the comparison. Other aspects may also need to be taken into account, such as how common a particular type of tool is considered to be, or the quantities that mass produced items are made in and how widely distributed they are.

Often the limiting factor in a marks' comparison is the quality of the scene mark. Detail that may be present on a tool may not be replicated in a mark for many reasons, such as the physical properties of the substrate. If it is only slightly softer than the tool the detail of interest may not be replicated in full.

If the substrate is very soft then it may be extensively damaged and, in the case of paint, may become smeared and any detail is obscured. If the surface of the substrate is textured it may interfere with any detail left by the tool or at the very least make it difficult for the examiner to reliably identify the important detail left by the tool.

The comparison of tool marks, and marks in general, is still a subjective area of forensic science, but there is an expectation by the courts that there is consistency amongst experts. It is therefore important to recognise that all experts must have knowledge of the relevant manufacturing processes, use the appropriate equipment and techniques to maximize the visualisation of the detail and have the skills and experience to undertake an examination. In any subjective examination difference of opinions will occasionally occur. The difference may only be slight and may be due to the difference in experience between the two experts. However, occasionally the difference will be significant and on occasions may even be to the extent that one expert will say the tool was responsible and the other that it was not the tool. With this in mind, the importance of an independent critical findings check by a second tool mark expert should not be underestimated. However, this is not always sufficient and a third expert may be required to undertake a check to decide the debate.

1.4   Training requirements for examiners

There are certain qualities that help make a good marks' examiner and some of the more important ones include good pattern recognition, a logical and methodical approach to work, good manipulation skills and an eye for detail. However, the most important factor is good training and coaching by an experienced examiner. To become a competent tool mark examiner takes time and controlled exposure to tool mark cases (with trainees in the other areas of marks' training having the equivalent exposure to relevant cases), which normally are mock/dummy cases to begin with, but after the individual has demonstrated their ability they may become an assistant to an experienced colleague and shadow them for a period of time.

The academic qualifications required to become a forensic practitioner in marks will vary around the world. In some countries a degree is normally required before being employed, although there are many examples in the United Kingdom where individuals have shown their expertise over a number of years as an examiner and have eventually been authorised to be a court reporting scientist. It may be useful at this point to clarify what is meant by a forensic examiner and a court reporting scientist. The court reporting scientist is the person with responsibility for planning the examination, evaluating the findings, writing the final statement and presenting the evidence in court if required as the expert witness. A forensic examiner is a person who is deemed technically competent to undertake the examination and comparison, which could be the court reporting scientist or another trained individual.

Tool mark examinations and the other related examinations that will be covered in this book, are not always undertaken by the same individuals or groupings of individuals. In some countries, such as the United States, tool marks are routinely done alongside firearms' and ballistics' work. It could be said that ballistics is a specific example of a tool mark as it involves consideration of the same types of class, sub-class and characteristic detail, often using the same comparison microscopes. With plastic packaging materials the expertise may reside within a drugs' department, as this is where the plastic materials are most frequently encountered. In our experience, marks' and traces' work is frequently encountered together and therefore physical scientists and chemists may work closely together. Here we mean 'traces' to be particulate in nature (rather than biological), which may require chemical, as well as microscopic, analysis, such as paint recovered from tools.

It is our view that the best and most successful approach to training examiners in tool marks or manufacturing marks is to develop a modular approach. A training course should identify the skills and knowledge required and must be tailored to achieve this desired outcome, in assessed stages where the scientist is deemed competent before proceeding. For example, in a traditional laboratory set-up where examiners and court reporting scientists work on cases together, it would not be necessary to train an examiner in all aspects of interpretation and evaluation. However, it would be necessary to train a reporting scientist in the technical aspects of examination. Each module should have an expected standard to be passed. For example, with casting techniques it would be expected that casting would be carried out to replicate the maximum detail with minimal air bubbles. It is recommended that an examiner becomes a competent microscopist, as this is a key aspect of most examinations.

Once each stage of the training programme has been passed and competency gained in each particular skill, then there should also be a programme in place to assess ongoing competency. Proficiency tests could be used for this purpose. These are set exercises that are focused on one particular aspect of the job and can be carried out on a regular basis. Training records should be kept, which are contemporaneous and demonstrate initial and ongoing competency.

The book does not provide a training programme as the authors recognise that one programme will not address everyone's needs and may not be appropriate for all organisations. However it is hoped that the content and discussion within the various chapters will provide a structure that identifies the competencies, skills, knowledge and experience required by a practitioner to undertake the work to the level of an expert.

1.5　Good forensic practice

It has been identified in many countries that there is an expectation by the general public, as well as the courts, that an expert witness will perform their work to a certain standard and behave in a certain way that meets the requirements of the legal system. In some cases these have been stated, an example being the UK Forensic Science Regulator's *Codes of Practice and Conduct* (2011). There are also other documents that provide guidance as to what is expected from an expert, for example, *The Criminal Procedure Rules* (Ministry of Justice, 2012).

Certainly within the United Kingdom (Association of Forensic Science Providers, *Standards for the Formulation of Evaluative Forensic Science Expert Opinion*, 2009) it is useful to try and ensure that any evidence that is presented is:

- logical

- transparent

- balanced

- robust.

In any forensic discipline it should be remembered that it is essential to ensure that good forensic practice is followed and for this area of forensic science it is no different. The application of sound principles of forensic conduct with regards to these examination types must be undertaken in a way that recognises the following.

- The importance of the chain of continuity from the crime scene to the court.

- The integrity of the any item being examined must be maintained.

- The potential of contamination occurring and steps taken to minimize the risk. This will include using the correct packaging and the protection, removal and retention of other significant forensic evidence such as fingerprints, DNA and other trace material.

- Any examination undertaken has to be scientifically valid and an examination should not be undertaken without the scientist understanding what is being compared and what the findings really mean.

- Only validated techniques are used in the examination. This is to say that any equipment or technique has been shown to be suitable and to produce the expected results/findings. Also, that the examiner is aware of the limitations or any critical settings of the equipment.

1.6   Examination and comparison strategy

In the following chapters of this book the examination and comparison of marks to tools is covered in depth; however, it is useful to summarise the strategy used in any comparison at this point as it establishes the approach that is taken. When dealing with any case there are a number of stages that are part of the examination process and should be considered by the practitioner, as follows.

1. Essential background information about the type of crime and any eyewitness account or other information that may be of use.

2. Location, enhancement and recovery from the crime scene – the crime scene examiner can provide significant information regarding the scene including the location of the mark(s).

3. Submission to the laboratory. Four stages of examination, which can be covered by a term used to describe the methodology for the examination of friction ridge detail in latent fingerprints '**ACE-V**' (SWGFAST, 2011):

    (a) **A**nalysis

    (b) **C**omparison

    (c) **E**valuation

    (d) **V**erification

1.6.1   Analysis

Analysis is the assessment of a tool mark (or material that can be considered to be 'unknown') to determine suitability for comparison. Factors considered include the following.

- Assessment of the information supplied and the question being asked by the submitting authority, whether or not there is any other information required before commencing.

- Assessment of material that has been supplied and if there any other considerations, such as the recovery of DNA, fingerprints or other trace materials.

- Development of an examination strategy derived from an assessment of what detail is present and how it should be enhanced to visualise it more clearly.

- Deciding what test marks are required.

1.6.2   Comparison

Comparison is the direct side by side observation of the relevant detail of interest to determine whether or not the detail is in agreement or different. This process will also involve interpretation of what the detail is and how it came to be present on the surface of the tool.

1.6.3   Evaluation

Evaluation is the formulation of a conclusion, based upon analysis and comparison of the relevant detail, by weighing up what the findings mean with respect to the prosecution and defence arguments. This will be covered in more detail in Chapter 6.

1.6.4   Verification

Verification is the independent examination by another qualified examiner. In any subjective marks' area within forensic science it is important that there is a final step in the process, which critically reviews the findings, the verification stage. This may also be known as a 'critical findings check'.

The verification process should ensure that:

- The examiner has followed the appropriate documented examination process and applied the appropriate and relevant scientific methodology and techniques.

- The work and findings of the examination are reflected in the conclusion reported. The results must support the conclusion and clearly there should be no understatement or overstatement of the findings.

- The maximum evidence has been obtained, that nothing has been overlooked and there are no other marks that may change the outcome.

- The submitting authority's question has been fully addressed.

1.7 Environment and equipment

Tool mark examinations are best carried out in a suitable environment, with appropriate equipment available for use. Although it is acknowledged that this will not always be possible, we will try to summarise a desirable environment in which to carry out laboratory examinations.

Throughout this book, reference may be made to 'laboratory examinations'. This is to make a distinction from 'scene examination', which may or may not be carried out by different individuals. However, it is recognised that some practitioners of marks' examinations do not strictly carry out their work in a laboratory as such (meaning either a room designed as a laboratory, or a wider organisation such as a forensic provider), although we would recommend this, as a stricter framework of protocol with respect to many aspects of the forensic process can be applied, controlled and monitored.

1.7.1 Basic requirements

A workbench or desk, preferably with good overhead lighting and an easily cleaned top, is required for the initial examination. Good health and safety procedures and anti-contamination procedures should be followed so the bench should also have electrical sockets placed so that equipment cables do not foul the working surface and allow for proper cleaning of the surface. The working surface needs to be cleaned before starting the examination. A further sensible precaution is to cover the work surface before starting the examination with a sheet of heavy paper, such as brown wrapping paper (also referred to as Kraft paper), which can be obtained in large rolls.

The workbench should be provided with a stereomicroscope with a magnification range of around times 8 to 30. The optics for the microscope needs a long working length (i.e. long focal length) and a good depth of field. The microscope should be mounted on a long arm microscope stand and have a flexible light source that can provide directional lighting rather than a ring source.

It is useful to have secondary light source available, fibre optics are often employed here, as they can be used for other examinations than tool marks.

1.7.2 Examiner's 'toolbox'

The examiner will need some hand tools; these can either be part of the bench equipment or part of the examiner's personal kit. A minimum list comprises a solid ruler, whose calibration can be traced back to a recognised authority, a flexible steel ruler, a knife or scalpel (scalpel blades can be disposed of to prevent contamination), scissors, tweezers and a probe (preferably with disposable needles). A hand lens with a magnification between times four and eight can also be useful. Vernier calipers (again with a traceable calibration) can help when measuring cylindrical objects. A chinagraph pencil can also be useful for marking tyres, for example.

Equipment to record the examination is needed; the main record is often on loose sheets of A4 paper held in a binder labelled with a reference given by the laboratory or by the submitting organisation. The A4 sheets are often pro formas, as there is standard information to be entered on each sheet, such as the type of item being examined and the item's reference, the date of the examination and the signature of the examiner(s). Many organisations also require the sheets to be numbered to ensure that none have been lost, which entails producing an index at the end of the examination. All entries on these sheets must be in ink and, where an alteration is needed, the text to be altered is lightly crossed through, so that it is still legible, the emendation made and initialled. Time can be saved by using a digital camera to record items and keep written descriptions to a minimum.

Other equipment that should be easily available is self-adhesive tape of different widths for repackaging exhibits, protective gloves and cleaning materials for the work surface. It is useful to have a waste bin, preferably with a foot-operated lid, close to the work bench.

1.7.3 Test mark and casting materials

When making a test mark with a submitted tool the examiner is trying to replicate the scene mark so that detail is reproduced and a comparison is possible. In most cases more than one test mark will have to be made so it is very important to use materials that do not change the detail that already exists on a tool or introduces new additional features. Therefore, the range of materials that are routinely used to undertake tool mark examinations includes: lead sheet and rod, modelling/dental wax and painted wood. On occasions it is necessary to use samples of the submitted material or even use the submitted item, a good example being plastic cable that has been cut. Other materials that it may be useful to have access to include those that will make the production, labelling and manipulation of casts produced in the laboratory easier, such as disposable paint brushes, backing paper and small wooden sticks such as toothpicks and lolly sticks.

The basic approach that has been developed over the past 20 plus years has been to develop procedures that enable the microscopic detail to be visualised and compared. Therefore, the development and improvement in microscopic equipment led to an increased use of casting materials. Many of these materials were originally designed for dental use but found an application in tool mark examination; in more recent years others have been specifically developed or modified for use in the forensic environment. So the use of casting materials has increased significantly not only to recover marks from a crime scene but also within the laboratory.

There are, however, a number of features that any material should have before it can be considered for routine use. It is recommended by the authors that any material that is being considered should be tested and validated for use. The important parameters that should be included in any assessment of a casting material are:

- dimensional stability over a long period of time;

- ability to capture and replicate very fine detail on the scale of microns;

- setting/curing characteristics;

- ease of use (includes mixing of the material to ensure all of the material hardens and removal from the mark without causing damage so that further casting is possible if needed);

- inert to a range of substrates;

- appearance under the microscope (opaque and not translucent);

- the ability to cast and recast the mark using another casting material but without loss of any detail.

Most of the current materials meeting these requirements are based on silicone rubbers. There are a number of sources for these, specialist stockists of scene of crime examination materials, engineering suppliers, jewellery equipment suppliers and dental supply houses.

There is a range of silicone rubbers that will meet the requirements above. The choice will depend on other local demands. Two-pack systems comprising base and hardener are the most flexible but need both experience

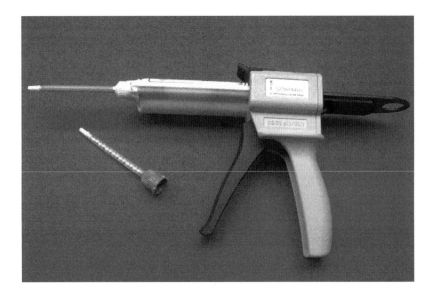

Figure 1.1   A single-pack system for casting.

and practice to use effectively. Thoroughly mixing the hardener with the base without introducing significant bubbles needs practice. In a single-pack system, depressing the plunger automatically mixes the base and hardener in the correct proportions in the disposable nozzle (Figure 1.1). These are far easier to use but care is needed in selecting the correct type for the conditions involved. In cold conditions, such as outdoor marks in winter, a quicker setting variety is needed than for the warmer conditions indoors or in summer. With two-pack systems the amount of hardener can be varied to take account of the temperature. Shelf life is also a consideration; when the silicone rubber no longer cures in the recommended time the pack must be thrown away; it should always be tested for setting time before use. With a two-pack system, using a fresh batch of hardener will often solve the problem.

Other casting materials have been used and references to these can be found in books, especially in older books such as *Crime Investigation* by Kirk (1953) or *Forensic Science* by Walls (1968). Some of these would no longer be acceptable, such as dental plaster or plasticine. Others, known generically as 'moulage', could still be used, provided that they are dimensionally stable and reproduce fine detail. They all suffer from the same problem, that they are mobile liquids when applied and thus require a containing wall to be built round the mark. This is best done with self-adhesive aluminium tape or plasticine; in fact, this technique can be useful even when using a silicone rubber.

The following list of casting materials is not comprehensive and is based on the authors' experience. Other materials are available and it is always worth experimenting to determine if there are better options. The list is in alphabetical order of the trade names that the materials are sold by.

- **Isomark**™: This silicone material is sold in a number of different grades, which cure at different rates. It is normally sold in cartridges that are used with an applicator 'gun', which mixes the base and hardener as the material is extruded through a nozzle. The quicker setting thixotropic materials work well in vertical or overhead marks, which make them especially useful for casting scene marks. It can bond to some materials, such as plastics or rubber, and should be tested on a small area of the substrate bearing the mark before use if there is any doubt regarding its ease of removal after curing. The slower curing, more fluid, grades are useful for casting horizontal, large areas of mark or deeply recessed ones.

- **Mikrosil**™: This a two-pack silicone system, comprising a base and hardener, that is mixed as needed. Some experience of the system is needed but it can be used in a wide variety of situations, both at a crime scene and in the laboratory.

- **Permlastic**™: This is a two-pack material, the base comprising a polysulfide material, which is used by dentists to recast from silicone rubbers. It is incompatible with Isomark casting material, on which it does not cure properly, but it can be used to recast from other silicone rubbers. It is not the best material for taking primary casts, as it is not very fluid, but can be used as an intermediary when making recasts from silicone rubber casts, for making replicas of metal tool parts or where the examination involves the physical fit of one part to another. Casts made with Permlastic will degrade in a relatively short time and are not suitable for long term storage.

- **Silcoset**™: This trade name covers a wide variety of products. The two of interest here are Silcoset 105 and Silcoset 101, whose primary listed purpose is for encapsulating items, with casting being a secondary use. They are both two-pack materials and a number of curing agents are suggested; for tool mark work the tin-based condensation curing agent is to be preferred.

- **Silmark**™: Similar to Mikrosil in that it is a two-pack system.

1.7.4 Larger equipment

In many tool mark cases, the detail that is compared is microscopic and can only be viewed on equipment that allows the detail to be resolved and visualised by the examiner. One of the most important aspects is to have lighting that allows the examiner to have complete control of the angle and direction of the light. In an ideal world, all examiners involved in tool mark work would have up-to-date comparators, but this is not always the case. Many examiners have to use old equipment and old lighting, which can limit the type of detail that can be compared. Other techniques have been utilised in the past and these have mainly been photographic based, but this approach is specialised and does have limitations.

1.7.4.1 The comparator   In essence an optical comparator comprises two microscopes that are joined by a bridge that allows the user to view both sample images side by side (Figure 1.2). The key parts of the instrument are the objective lenses. As the samples will be viewed in reflected light, the lens needs to have a working distance that is as large as possible to allow for effective lighting. Additionally, the lens needs the numerical aperture to be as small as possible to give a good depth of field. Both of these requirements are best met with objectives giving low magnifications.

Owing to the comparison aspect of the work, there is a very important factor that must be considered, no matter what equipment or method is being used to undertake the comparison. There is a need to ensure that one is comparing like with like. This means that the equipment is balanced and calibrated so that the examiner can establish the magnification and also be confident that when detail is different or when it matches it is an accurate reflection and not an artefact due to an error in the set-up of the equipment.

A pair of calibrated scaled graticules can be used for this purpose (Figure 1.3). Depending on the comparator model being used and the protocols adopted, these are used to check the balance of the comparator prior to use. A record should be kept in the notes and in auditable written/computer records relating to the comparator when this is done. Some models of comparators will also have a light to indicate that they are balanced, but these should still have the balance checked periodically to ensure that it has not drifted and to show that the equipment is working properly.

This raises the question of what is the useful range of magnification required for a detailed tool mark examination? For most comparisons, objective lenses with magnifications in the range of from ×0.5 to ×20 with ×10 eyepieces should suffice. As the total magnification is objective × eyepiece this would give a range of ×5 to ×200. If the detail to be examined is in the millimetre to centimetre size range, then it becomes more difficult to obtain a large enough field of view with a microscope to show all the detail at the same time. However, with modern equipment it is possible to view the mark in sections and stitch together the images to show the entire mark. In some cases macro photography may be more useful. Detail smaller than a few microns (i.e. 1×10^{-3} mm) in size may be very variable and hard to reproduce in test marks. However, if the tool used has a reasonably reproducible action (such as a

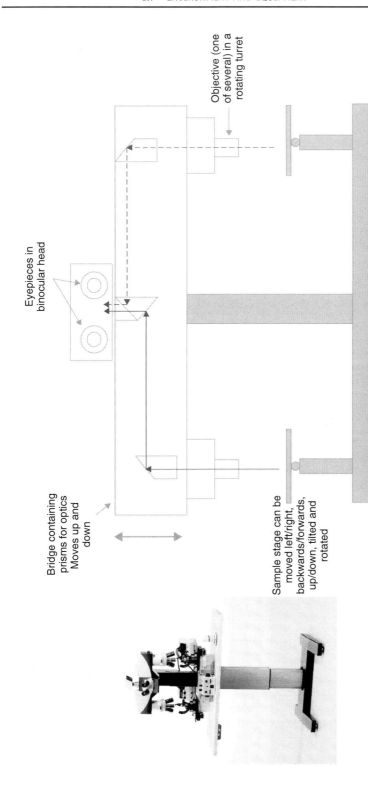

Objective (one of several) in a rotating turret

Eyepieces in binocular head

Bridge containing prisms for optics Moves up and down

Sample stage can be moved left/right, backwards/forwards, up/down, tilted and rotated

Figure 1.2 A comparator, set up for an examination of two bullets, is shown on the left (© Leica). A specimen holder is not usually required for tool mark purposes and fibre optic lighting is preferred. These alterations can be made to the general set up, as shown in Figure 1.4. A schematic diagram of how light passes through a comparator is shown on the right.

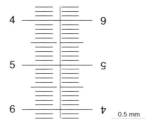

Figure 1.3 A balance check using scaled graticules, shows that the comparator is balanced as the scales line up exactly.

stapler or double bladed cutter) a series of test marks may be able to capture suitable detail. If necessary, it is possible to cast this detail and visualise it using a scanning electron microscope (SEM) rather than an optical comparator. Thus, detail at this level should not be ignored, but may be difficult to compare.

If the higher total magnifications, say from ×100 to ×200, are to be used then there may be problems due to building vibrations. Nearly all building structures have vibrations present, from wind pressure or traffic, if no other cause. The vibrations result in problems for the comparator, as the objective lenses are mounted some distance apart on the optical bridge, which allows the objectives to vibrate independently. At low total magnifications this is not very important, but it can result in image degradation at higher total magnifications. The severity of the problem will dictate what will need to be done, but it can easily be addressed by using a heavy table or some type of damping system, such as an anti-vibration mat. If the vibration problem is indeed significant, then some form of anti-vibration system is needed; complex systems, such as those used for laser optics may be required.

A number of different item stages are available for comparators. For tool marks the stages need to have three-dimensional (x, y and z) adjustment and have a rotatable stage head. This means that the stage can be moved smoothly to left and right (x axis), forwards and backwards (y axis) and up and down (z axis), as well as being rotated. In addition, it should be possible to tilt the stage with respect to the optic axis of the objective lens. This implies that there is some type of universal, or ball, joint just below the stage head and before the stage links into the x, y and z adjustments. It is possible to use a plastic material, such as plasticine or Blu-Tack™, to attach the item to the comparator stage and this can be used to orient the item with respect to the optic axis but, by itself, this may cause problems in obtaining the best illumination of the item that is to be examined. A tilting stage head can help overcome this problem.

In the process of comparing the mark, the stage needs to be moved in the $x–y$ plane and this makes it necessary to have the lighting system attached to the stage (Figure 1.4), so that a constant level of illumination is maintained. The lights may be either independent or a single source with fibre optics to

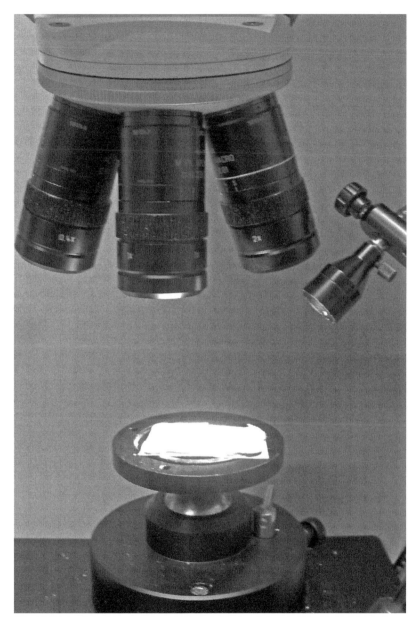

Figure 1.4 A tool mark cast illuminated on a comparator stage. For most tool mark examinations the light will normally be at a shallow angle, rather than at 45° as shown here.

bring the light to each stage. In either case, the light beam produced should be as near parallel as possible. Single source lighting has some advantages if the comparator is to be used with camera systems. The single light source removes some of the problems involved with obtaining balanced light through both objective lenses, although modern lights are often much better in terms of balanced light. Some older models of comparator also have a focusing adjustment to narrow or widen the beam of light. However, more modern models do not.

Some laboratories have utilised features of the SEM as a specialised imaging and comparison tool (Sehgal *et al*, 1988), in some instances using a pair of SEMs to undertake the comparison (Katterwe *et al*, 1982). Each instrument is used to image the detail of interest and to compare the images produced side by side on the screen of the instrument. Otherwise individual screen images are printed and the printed images used for the comparison. In these cases, it is important to have a scale printed in with the image.

1.8 Quality assurance

In addition to having a verification process, there are various ways that forensic providers, individuals or organisations, can provide quality assurance to their customers and ultimately to the Criminal Justice System.

The UK Home Office's appointment of a Forensic Science Regulator in 2007/2008 was a step towards establishing and maintaining quality standards in line with ISO 17025 and European Union law, in a much more fragmented forensic market place, where, since the closure of the Forensic Science Service in 2012, there are now multiple private providers working alongside in-house police laboratories. The Forensic Science Regulator has produced a document called *Codes of Practice and Conduct* (2011), which details what is expected of all forensic providers and practitioners.

In the United Kingdom, the ultimate aim for organisations would be to gain the accreditation ISO 17025 via The United Kingdom Accreditation Service (UKAS) who are working very closely with the Forensic Science Regulator. It is acknowledged that this may be a much more difficult and lengthy process for smaller laboratories. A laboratory applying for this accreditation would have to show that they meet the required standards. The standards include:

- that there are up-to-date, controlled procedures documented for the work being carried out,

- that everyone who is doing this type of work has been trained and is competent to do so.

ISO 17025 provides a comprehensive international standard covering various areas that need to be addressed, including management structure, procedures and processes as well as technical requirements, such as training and equipment.

To begin at the beginning then, it is important to have scientific procedures documented and also to have training and on-going competency programmes in place. This will ensure that everyone carrying out the work is doing it to the required standard, following procedures, in a consistent manner.

There is an expectation that any organisation will be able to provide evidence that there is control regarding the quality of work being delivered. There are various approaches to demonstrating that work is being delivered consistently and to the standard required, and these include assessing a randomly selected sample of practitioners' cases against specific criteria (also known as 'dip' checks), method audits, competency tests, declared and undeclared trials.

It is less easy to regulate the training and competency of forensic experts who work alone. However, at the very least one would expect an 'expert' to carry out work within their acknowledged area of expertise and in accordance with a written code of practice. There have been some attempts to introduce regulation into the forensic field as a whole, to assure the courts and the general public that experts in court were indeed qualified experts who were trained, with sufficient experience of the subject matter to be able to offer a considered opinion. However, these attempts have been limited in terms of their impact thus far. For those experts working within an accredited organisation, this should go without saying, as they are regulated by their company and its accreditation process.

1.9 A brief summary

It is the authors' intentions in this book to provide those interested in this area of forensic science with the essential principles and knowledge required to carry out examinations of this type. We hope that the preceding information has been sufficient to give the reader a flavour of the basic foundations of marks' examinations that a would-be practitioner would have to consider before embarking on work of this nature. Clearly, amongst other prerequisites, there is a requirement for any practitioner to gain expertise in the use of the instrumentation available to them, which is fundamental to the visualisation of detail required for a meaningful comparison. To obtain the best results, this equipment should ideally be similar to that described in this book.

Whilst we hope that this book can provide guidance and clarity over the areas required to gain expertise in this interesting field of forensic work, it should not be seen as providing all the information on all aspects of it. However, hopefully, the contents will encourage greater understanding, perhaps raising some interesting discussion points amongst those involved in the various areas of work discussed, to aid development in this field.

References

Association of Forensic Science Providers (2009) Standards for the formulation of evaluative forensic science expert opinion. *Science and Justice*, **49** (3), 161–164.

Biasotti, A.A. (1964) The principles of evidence evaluation as applied to firearms and tool mark identification. *Journal of Forensic Sciences*, **9** (4), 428–433.

Davis, J.E. (1958) *An Introduction to Toolmarks, Firearms and the Striagraph*, Charles C. Thomas, Springfield, Illinois.

Forensic Science Regulator (2011) *Codes of Practice and Conduct for Forensic Science Providers and Practitioners in the Criminal Justice System*. Crown Copyright 2011, Version 1.0, December.

Gross, H. (1893) *Handbuch für Untersuchungsrichter als System der Kriminalistik. Polizeibeamte, Gendarmen, usw*, Leutzner und Lubowsky, Graz.

Gross, H. (1907) *Criminal Investigation: A Practical Textbook for Magistrates, Police Officers and Lawyers*, (translated by J. Adam and J. Collyer Adam), Lawyers' Co-Operative Publishing, New York.

Katterwe, H., Goebel, R. and Grooss, K.D. (1982) The comparison scanning electron microscope within the field of forensic science. *Scanning Electron Microscopy*, Part 2, 499–504.

Kirk, P.L. (1953) *Crime Investigation: Physical Evidence and the Police Laboratory*, Interscience Publishers Inc., New York.

Ministry of Justice (2012) *The Criminal Procedure Rules*. Crown Copyright, http://www.justice.gov.uk/courts/procedure-rules/criminal/rulesmenu (accessed October 2012).

Sehgal, V.N., Singh, S.R., Dey, A., *et al.* (1988) Tool marks comparison of a wire cut ends by scanning electron microscopy – A forensic study. *Forensic Science International*, **36** (1–2), 21–29.

SWGFAST (Scientific Working Group on Friction Ridge Analysis, Study and Technology) (2011) *Standards for Examining Friction Ridge Impressions and Resulting Conclusions*. Version 1.0. www.swgfast.org/Documents.html (accessed October 2012).

Walls, H.J. (1968) *Forensic Science: An Introduction to Scientific Crime Detection*, Sweet & Maxwell Ltd, London.

2
Tool Manufacture

2.1 Introduction

Tools are implements that help a person to carry out a particular, usually legitimate, task. In terms of criminal offences, however, the action with which the tool is used may vary from that originally intended (but nonetheless help an offender to achieve their goal). For example, a screwdriver could be used to lever apart two objects such as a window and a frame rather than to screw in a screw, or a kitchen knife could be used to stab a tyre or a person rather than for culinary purposes. It is unsurprising then that tool marks can be found in a wide variety of substrates in offences ranging from criminal damage and burglary to murder and terrorist cases.

Many types of hand tool are easily accessible and portable and therefore more frequently encountered in forensic examinations than larger, more cumbersome tools and machinery. Levering and cutting tools such as screwdrivers, case openers[1] (Figure 2.1) and bolt cutters are the most notable of those seen during the collective working careers of the authors; however, there may be variations in the type and frequency of the tools seen if there are particular crime trends occurring in an area of the country, such as locking pliers[2] being used to break EuroProfile™ style locks. Other, more specialist, tools such as an embossing machine used in a fraud case, may be seen rarely.

In all cases though, it is the shape, size and surface features of the contact areas of the tool that may be left in a substrate, which can then be used

---

[1] The term 'case opener' is used generically here to mean tools such as wrecking bars, crowbars, pry bars, Gorilla™ bars and the like. These are sometimes also known as 'jemmies' (or 'jimmies' in the United States), although this term could be considered to be pejorative as it often refers specifically to tools used to break into premises.
[2] Such as Mole Grips™ or Vise Grips™.

The Forensic Examination and Interpretation of Tool Marks, First Edition.
David Baldwin, John Birkett, Owen Facey and Gilleon Rabey.
© 2013 John Wiley & Sons, Ltd. Published 2013 by John Wiley & Sons, Ltd.

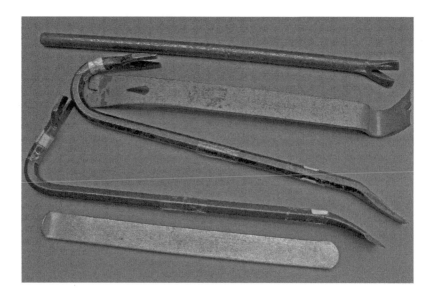

Figure 2.1   A collection of case openers and a tyre lever.

for comparison purposes. Surface features can be microscopic or large in nature and can include those left during manufacture of the tool or those formed subsequently on it during the tool's use or misuse. These features are sometimes called class, sub-class or individual features/characteristics depending on how they were produced.

Class features are those that have been determined prior to production of a particular tool, such as the type and action of the tool or its size. Sub-class features are similar markings that have been produced on some or all of a run of tools from a particular mould or machine, which could be an intended feature, such as pressed lines, or an incidental one such as damage to the mould. Individual characteristics are as the name suggests. They are unique to a tool and have been randomly acquired as the tool is used and becomes worn and damaged or through a manufacturing process, such as grinding.

It would be very unusual for a newly made tool not to show any sort of surface detail. Many tools will undergo some sort of finishing process, either to give a pleasing aesthetic look or to give the tool its main function, such as to form a cutting edge. In addition, tools nearly always suffer minor, microscopic damage during the manufacturing process, handling and storage, which gives them individual character.

Given the large variety of tools available, which require different properties depending on their intended use, it is little wonder that there is huge variation in the processes used in the production of tools. Tools of the same type and size, but produced by different tool companies, may have an entirely different final appearance and finish, depending on the combination of manufacturing

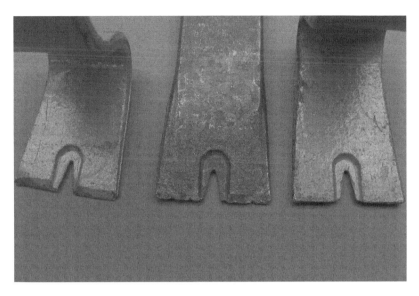

Figure 2.2 Three pry bars, with a plain bevel (left), ground bevel (middle) and no bevel (right).

and finishing processes used. Figure 2.2 shows the working ends of three pry bars, one of which has a plain bevel (left), a ground bevel (middle) and no bevel (right). Even within the same company, a budget and a quality range of tools of the same type and size may be produced, with different specifications and finishes. In addition, some tools that are produced abroad may be finished in the United Kingdom for sale there. Some manufacturers may simply apply their brand labelling to the tools before sale, but others may go further by grinding off any imperfections and applying their brand's paint colour.

You will not always know exactly how a particular tool has been produced from start to finish, unless it is clearly branded and the manufacturer's process has been investigated. In many tool mark cases this course of action would be unnecessary as it may not be relevant to the tool mark under examination, or there may be more distinguishing features present on the tool, such as damage, which would supersede any manufacturing detail, if found in the mark. However, there should be clues on the tool's surface to help you decide how it was made.

This chapter will therefore aim to provide an overview only of some of the main processes involved in tool production that a forensic tool mark examiner should be aware of, concentrating more on those that create surface features on a tool. More detailed information concerning the production of particular types of tools, such as saws, will be given later on in this book where relevant, mainly in Chapters 4 and 5. With a good awareness of the types of manufacturing features that can be found on the surface of a tool, an examiner should be able to apply that knowledge to the examination of a tool that they have never seen before or is not discussed here. Surface features formed during use and potential interpretation issues will also be discussed.

2.2   Working with metal

Tools need to be hardwearing and able to cope with the stresses and strains placed upon them during manufacture and use. Metal is ideal for this purpose. The working parts of tools are usually formed from the alloy steel, which is mainly made up of iron with lesser amounts of carbon and other non-metallic and/or metallic elements added. The composition of the steel can be varied depending on the desired properties for the tool, such as corrosion resistance or increased strength. Steel is usually available in various forms as a stock material for tool production: coils of thick 'wire' (which we will refer to as 'rod' once cut to size to form the shafts of screwdrivers and similar), bars, sheets, ingots, metal powders and so on.

Tool metals are often complex compounds that can be manipulated using temperature programs and force as needed during manufacture, to produce a tool of the appropriate shape with the properties required. When metal is shaped cold at room temperatures, usually with smaller tools such as some screwdrivers, it can make the metal more brittle and harder to work with (also known as 'work hardening'). However, this effect can be reversed by a heat treatment known as annealing. There are various methods of annealing, but in general the metal is heated to beyond its 'recrystallization temperature' (whereby internal stresses are relieved and its grain structure changes to a more stable state), then cooled gradually and slowly under controlled conditions, making the metal less brittle and easier to machine.

At high temperatures, that is, when the metal is heated to red hot in a furnace (Plate 1), metal can be bent and shaped more easily. This hot forging method would be more appropriate for chunkier pieces, such as a metal bar being shaped to form the curved ends of a wrecking bar. Because the metal is shaped whilst above its recrystallization temperature, annealing of the metal effectively takes place while the metal is being worked.

Hot metal items, following hot forging, are often quenched in cold water or oil to rapidly cool and harden them again, but this process can make the metal brittle and can produce surface scale in the presence of oxygen. With oil quenching the oil will need to be washed off as well. Tools that have been subjected to this sort of hardening need to be tempered (a type of annealing), where they are placed in a tempering oven at more moderate temperatures, which reduces stress. This hardening method can also be used with cold metal items such as screwdrivers. These would need to be heated in a furnace first, but can then be subjected to quenching, cleaning and tempering steps as described.

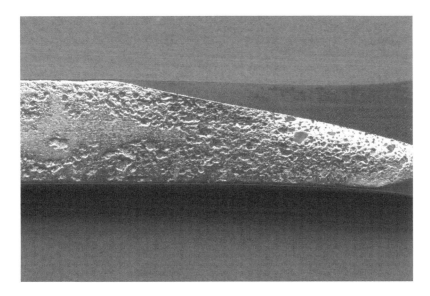

Figure 2.3 The rough, pitted surface of a hot forged tool.

The exact temperatures used in these techniques will vary depending on the composition of the metal and the desired results. Temperature differentials also need to be taken into account when working with metal. For example, a red-hot piece of metal being forged with a cold hammer and anvil could cause thermal shock in the metal, creating weak points and causing it to fail at a later stage. Equipment therefore also needs to be at the correct temperature.

This is just a brief overview of some of the hardening and heat treatments that tools may go through during manufacture. There are others, all of which will depend on the exact composition of the metal and outcome to be achieved. However, hardening and heat treatment is usually done at some point during the manufacturing process of every tool and may be done to all or part of the tool depending on the desired results. For example, it may be necessary to have a screwdriver with a particularly hardwearing tip or a case opener with some flexibility in the shaft. The metal surface could show irregularities from the underlying microscopic structure or from heat treatments (Figure 2.3).

2.3 Creating a tool 'blank'

In tool manufacture, usually a 'blank' is formed first from the stock material being used. This will be the rough shape of the tool being produced. This pre-forming of a tool can involve various metal shaping and cutting techniques, the majority of which will be described in this chapter. Finishing processes, by comparison, prepare the tool for sale and use, either to make it look aesthetically pleasing or to give it its main function, such as grinding an edge to sharpen it. Throughout its manufacture, a tool is usually referred to as the 'work piece' until it is finished. For some very cheap tools, creating a blank will be the only stage in producing the main body of a tool, but a handle may be added or components fitted together.

Creating a blank can be as simple as using a die and punch to cut a shape out of a flat sheet of metal, as with most saw blades or some cheaper quality knife blades. Steel wire can be straightened, cut or sawn to length and drawn to decrease the diameter; rods can be rolled to create bars with different cross-sections, forming shafts ready for forging. Sintering and casting can be used to create more complex shapes, which in both cases entail using a mould. In sintering, dry metal powder in the mould is heated and fused together. In casting, molten metal is poured into a mould and left to cool, after which the work piece can be removed.

2.3.1   Forging

Forging is the shaping of metal under the application of force at different temperatures. The traditional concept of a blacksmith using a hammer and anvil to shape metal is in no way obsolete, indeed some tools may still be produced entirely by hand in this way. However, in this age that requires high productivity, powered machinery is often used to aid the operator, or in the case of mass production, automated machinery can be used with minimal operator input.

Open and closed die drop forging are two methods that are often used in tool manufacture. Drop forging involves powered machinery consisting of a stationary anvil, onto which the work piece is placed, with a heavy hammer on a ram above. The powered ram is raised to lift the hammer, which is then dropped onto the work piece, administering a strike. If necessary, the ram can be lifted again to deliver repetitive strikes.

With open die forging, the surfaces of the hammer and anvil are usually flat and sometimes angled relative to each other, when required for the shape of the tool. A case opener blade is a good example of a tool requiring angled dies. As the hammer strikes up and down, the hot work piece is manipulated and turned by the operator (Plate 2). Other shaping techniques, such as bending the shaft of a case opener to form a swan neck (Plate 3) or creating the double bladed end, can be done whilst the metal is hot using special fixtures (Plate 4). Open die forging is sometimes also known as 'free hand' forging. The final shape and size can therefore vary slightly between pieces produced by the same or different operators.

Closed die forging reduces this sort of variation in class features. At least one of the plates, usually the anvil, has a mould (closed die) on it. There may be multiple moulds on the plate for successive shaping of the tool or there may be corresponding moulds on the top and bottom plates. In all cases, when the work piece is held in place over the mould and the hammer strikes it from above, the metal is forced to take the shape of the mould or moulds. Closed die forging can be used to make blanks for a wide range of tools, from those with shaped blades to axe and hammer heads to bolt cutter or plier jaws.

Any pattern or manufacturing detail in a die or mould will be transferred to subsequent work pieces produced in it. In addition, if that die or mould is damaged, the defect(s) could also be reproduced on each work piece produced by that equipment, whilst in that condition. These types of sub-class features can have implications for interpretation as more than one tool could potentially produce marks showing the same detail. If there was any grinding detail on the die or mould used in the forging process, this would be impressed onto the work piece and every tool made from those dies/moulds would have the same apparent grinding detail (but in 'negative') on them. The examiner would need to determine that this detail has, in fact, been impressed onto the tool and was not the result of direct grinding.

Another type of forging is known as upset forging, which occurs in a horizontal plane. The free end of a heated bar is punched or hammered, forcing the other end to either assume the shape of a cavity (such as with the formation of bolts) or to form a widened ball against a surface. This latter technique can be used when making flat bladed tools, such as brick bolsters, where the blade is integral with the shaft and will be significantly wider than the original bar stock. The ball at the end can then be flattened and shaped by a drop forging method (Plate 5).

2.3.2   Blanking and shearing

Blanking (also known as stamping) is one of the more commonly used methods that can be used to produce flat shaped work pieces out of metal strips and sheets. The metal sits on top of a die with a shaped hole in it and a correspondingly shaped punch is dropped from above. The punch passes into the die forcing the metal to go through with it as well. The metal shears and breaks off to produce the shaped piece in the die. The edge of the metal will show a rolled down top (where it has been stretched into the hole), then an area of burnishing followed by fracture and burring. A similar process can be used to create holes and other features where metal is removed from work pieces, generally known as punching (but with more specific names such as piercing, perforation and so on, depending on the desired results).

Shearing can occur in any process where two opposing forces pass each other through cold metal and the excess metal is clipped off. For example, some screwdriver blades are formed by first flattening the end of a steel rod, then placing this on a lower die, which is shaped like a screwdriver blade. A moving upper die cuts off the excess metal (Figures 2.4). This contrasts with hot closed die forged metal where excess metal squeezes out between

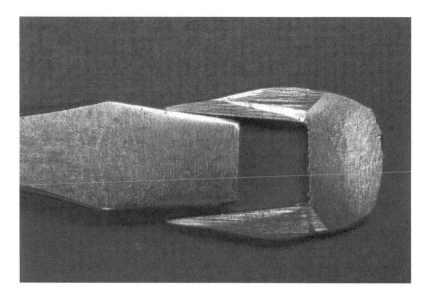

Figure 2.4 Excess metal clipped off a screwdriver blade.

two dies and does not break off. This is known as 'flash'. An example of flash, underneath the head of a nail, is shown in Chapter 7, Figure 7.3. Flash can be subsequently ground off or otherwise removed from a tool, as can shearing and fracture detail. However, sometimes these features may still be present on a tool under examination and could be evidentially significant. Caution should be taken with shearing detail, as this could appear similar on tools formed in the same equipment (Burd and Gilmore, 1968). However, as the microscopic structure of metal will be individual to the tool, one would expect fracture detail to be unique (Figure 2.5).

2.3.3 Metal cutting operations

Cross-head screwdrivers such as 'Phillips' are made from steel rod. The tip is cut to the correct angle first and then a grinding disc held perpendicular to the rod adds flutes. The rod is rotated in order to cut the next flute. A similar process can be used to produce the helical flutes on drill bits.

Milling is a metal cutting operation that can be used to shape work pieces or to create three-dimensional objects, such as moulds, from which other tools are produced. Milling marks are most often encountered in the laboratory on tools that have bevelled edges, such as bolt cutter and chisel blades (Figure 2.6). Milling is done using a cutter with a number of evenly spaced teeth. The work piece is moved past the rotating cutter, which produces evenly spaced, regular marks of similar height and width. The marks may appear straight and parallel or curved, depending on the method of milling,

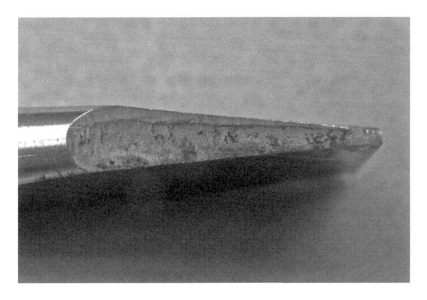

Figure 2.5 Sheared and fractured edge of a screwdriver blade.

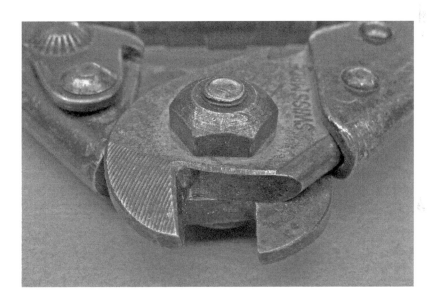

Figure 2.6 Milling marks on the top blade.

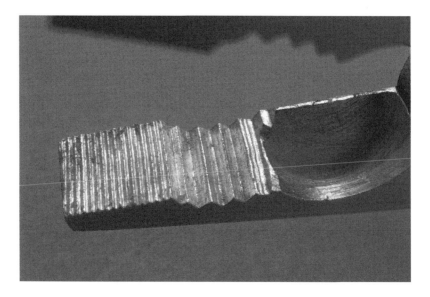

Figure 2.7   Broached teeth of a pair of pliers.

type of cutter used and size of the area of tool that has been milled. Milling can appear macroscopically similar on consecutively milled tools, especially when the milling marks are reproduced in a similar position in relation to the tip and/or an edge (Miller and Beach, 2005). Direct milling of a tool's surface results in milling with a crisp appearance. This compares to milling detail that has been replicated from the inside of a milled mould or die, where the detail on the tool's surface will not appear so crisp.

Broaching is another type of metal cutting operation, where serrated broaching tools are used to form the teeth of hand tools such as pliers and wrenches (Figure 2.7). Other metal cutting operations, such as those that can produce holes, may also be used in tool production; for example, pivot holes in bolt cutter blades may be drilled and reamed. However, these do not feature routinely in tool mark examinations and so will not be discussed further here.

2.4   Finishing processes

A variety of mechanical and chemical methods can be used at points during manufacture to degrease and clean work pieces, to remove oxidation products, scale, burrs or other unwanted effects formed during heat treatment, forging and cutting and to shine and polish. In one such method, work pieces are loaded into a drum or vat and tumbled or vibrated with an abrasive medium, water and chemicals to clean and polish them. The size and type of media together with added compounds can vary depending on what the desired result is. For example, ceramic pebbles, oxalic acid, polishing and anti-rust

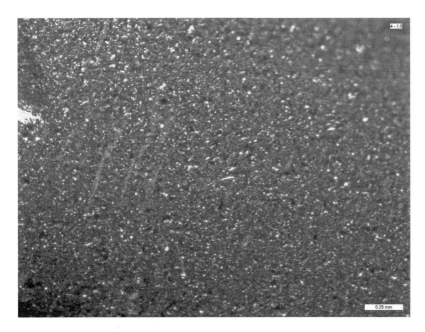

Figure 2.8 Shot-blasted tip of a cross-head screwdriver (very fine aluminium oxide particles used).

compounds could be used to clean and polish screwdrivers. In very small areas, such as the characters of metal stamps, scale may remain after cleaning.

Shot blasting is another method of cleaning and removing surface defects from a work piece, whilst giving a pleasing aesthetic finish. It can also be a finishing process in itself, done after plating, such as to the tips of screwdrivers. Shot blasting is a random process so the surface finish will be unique, particularly if no further processes are undertaken to change the work piece before the final tool is produced. The whole or part of the work piece can be bombarded with shot. For example, case openers may be entirely shot blasted while being held in the basket of a shot-blasting machine, whereas a screwdriver could be held in a rubber ferrule and the shot solely focused on the tip. Shot particles can vary in size from very fine grit to ball bearings, which will give a fine (Figure 2.8) to rough surface finish, respectively. Typically the shot needs to be harder than the work piece, for example, harder steel or aluminium oxide. Sand can also be used for cleaning, although this would not show as a noticeable texture on the metal surface.

At this point the 'work piece' has been formed into the basic tool with perhaps just a few extra processes being used to give the tool its final finished appearance. For simplicity, from this point on we will refer to the work piece as the tool.

Coatings, such as metallic plating or non-metallic paint and varnish, can also be applied to the surface of tools for reasons such as aestheticism and

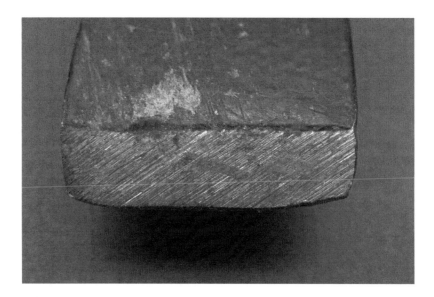

Figure 2.9   Paint ground off the tip of a tool, in order to add a bevel.

brand identification (in terms of paint colour), to help prevent wear or to aid corrosion resistance. Coatings could be applied to all or part of a tool and those coatings may be subsequently removed in part, for example, by grinding paint off the tip of a blade to form a bevel (Figure 2.9). Coatings can also be applied on top of grinding or other machine finishes.

Electroplating methods can be used to apply thin metallic coatings to cleaned, degreased tools. Chromium is commonly used to plate screwdriver shafts and blades. This does not adhere well directly to steel and so copper or nickel may be used as an intermediary coating. Screwdriver tips are often, but not always, left unplated as any flexing of the tip under high torque conditions could cause the hard chromium plating to flake off. Screwdrivers with plating on the tips can be found. Gripping tools such as locking pliers usually have plating on the jaws, including the gripping surface, which can chip off.

Grinding and linishing marks are commonly encountered on tools (Figures 2.10 and 2.11). Grinding and linishing are metal cutting operations. Some screwdriver blades are primarily produced by grinding a face into the end of a steel rod (Figure 2.12). However, these are mainly used as finishing techniques to remove flash, shearing and other unwanted detail from primary shaping and cutting processes. They can also be used to make a leading edge sharp and operable, or to bring a tool blade within certain size tolerances. In some instances, grinding or linishing may simply be done to provide a decorative finish, as the customers of a particular manufacturer may feel that it shows the tool has been properly finished (even if it is to the detriment of the tool's function, such as potentially leaving areas of weakness, prone to fracture).

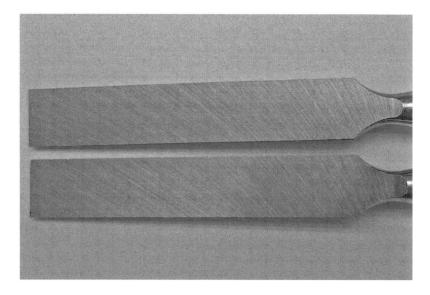

Figure 2.10 Grinding marks on the back surfaces of two wood chisels.

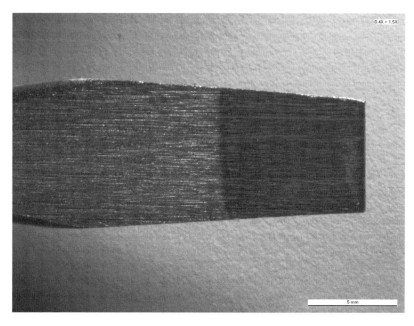

Figure 2.11 Linishing marks on a screwdriver blade. The tip has been heat treated to strengthen it.

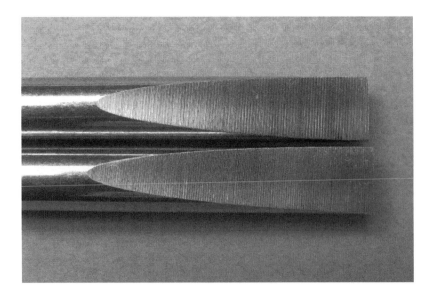

Figure 2.12   Screwdriver blades formed by grinding metal rod.

Tool production grinding can be done singly by hand on a grinding wheel or linishing belt (Figure 2.13). Batches of tools can have their faces and tips ground at the same time, by being clamped in a jig over a grinding wheel (Figure 2.14) or mounted on a magnetic rotary grinder. With the exception of tips being ground in an automated process, tips and edges of bladed tools are more often ground or linished by hand, which can introduce variation into individual blade dimensions as well as irregularity as described below.

In all of the above scenarios, grinding and linishing entails holding the tool against a moving abrasive surface. Generally the abrasive surface can be thought of as having multiple tiny cutting tools on it, which will leave a series of fine and/or coarse grooves on the surface of the tool. Abrasives used can range from ceramic grit on a linishing belt to carbide based grinding wheels with added chromium oxide for example. As the abrasive is used it will break down through wear and the grinding surface will change. More information on the mechanics of grinding is given in a paper by Monturo (2010). A paper about marks made by bolt cutters, by Butcher and Pugh (1975), describes grinding stones wearing down with use and needing to be redressed, with the period between redressing varying depending on how uneven the stone has become with use.

Depending on how the tool is held against the abrasive, grinding marks could run horizontally across the blade or longitudinally along the length of the blade. Linishing detail is usually longitudinal. A single tool could have grinding and/or linishing detail on its different sides (Figure 2.15), meeting at various angles on the edges, adding evidential significance to a comparison if

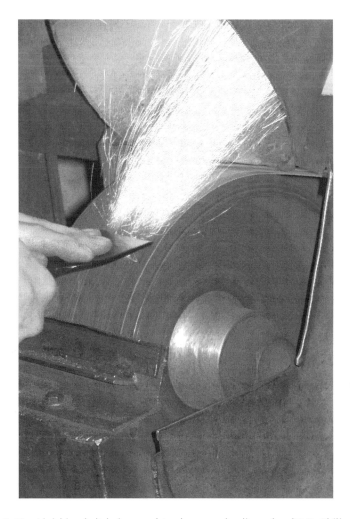

Figure 2.13 Linishing belt being used to sharpen a leading edge (© Dr Philip Davis).

found in a tool mark and on a tool or in test marks made by it (in the case of striated marks).

Hand grinding results in detail that does not reproduce on consecutively ground tools. This occurs because, for both the wheel and belt systems, the tool can initially be placed randomly on any part of the large, rotating grinding surface, at a range of angles both horizontally and vertically. In addition, as we have already seen, the character of the abrasive surface is constantly changing. All of these factors result in unique detail being produced on each tool ground using the equipment.

Simultaneous grinding detail can be a lot more regular as grooves produced by individual abrasive particles in the surface of one blade face can continue and follow onto the surface of one or more blade faces placed next to it.

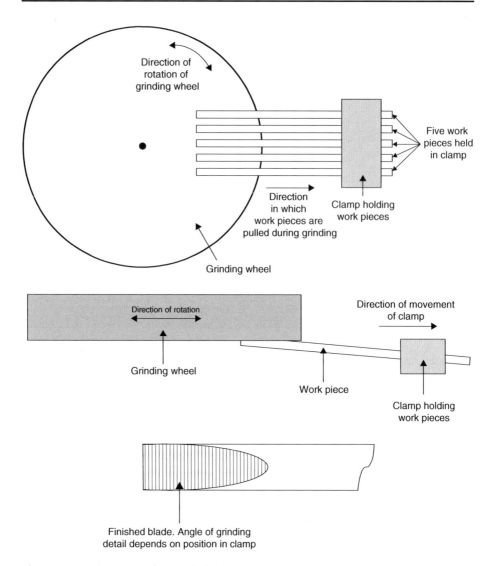

Figure 2.14   Diagram to show tools held in a clamp over a grinding wheel for simultaneous grinding. Side view (top), plan view (middle) and finished screwdriver blade after grinding (bottom).

Regular grinding can therefore look very similar between simultaneously ground tools, although the exact angle and curve of the grooves can vary in relation to the tip and edges. This is easy to see when simultaneously ground, adjacent blades are subsequently placed next to each other in order (Figure 2.16); however, given one such tool in isolation and a limited quality tool mark, it could be difficult to use the grinding detail alone as a distinguishing feature. Looking at adjacently ground blades, one may see

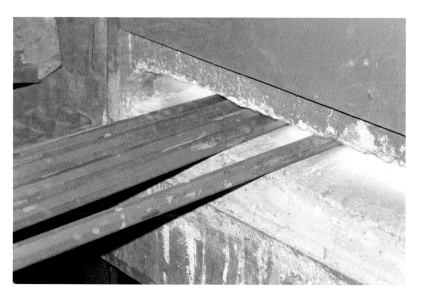

Plate 1 Metal bars being heated in a furnace (© Dr Philip Davis).

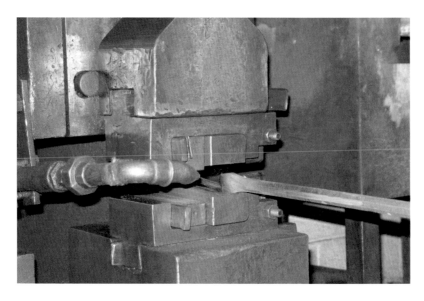

Plate 2   Open die drop forging the single bladed end of a case opener (© Dr Philip Davis).

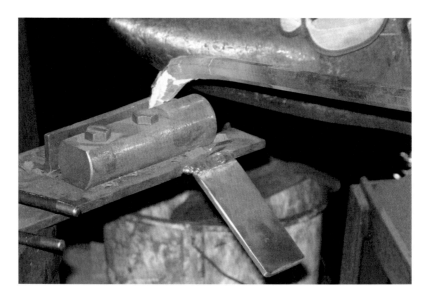

Plate 3   Bending a swan neck (© Dr Philip Davis).

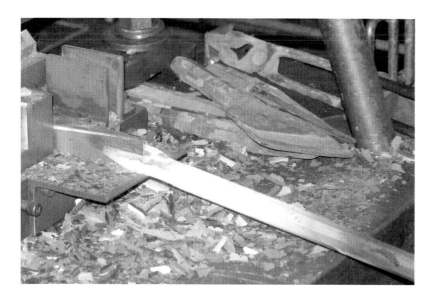

Plate 4 Using a cutting fixture to make a double blade (© Dr Philip Davis).

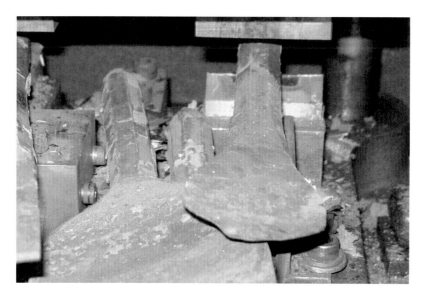

Plate 5 Ball end of an upset forged metal bar, flattened by drop forging (© Dr Philip Davis).

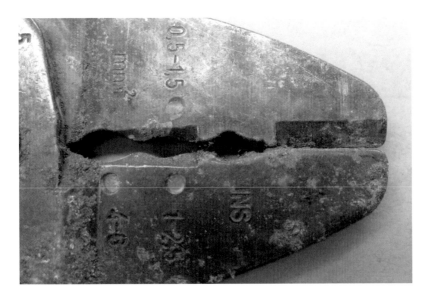

Plate 6 Corrosion giving a pitted appearance to parts of the tool's surface.

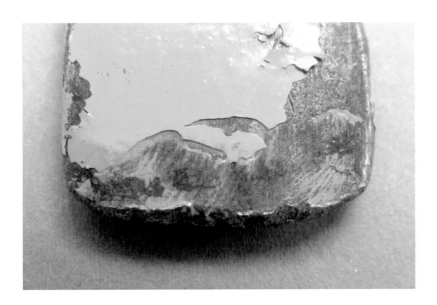

Plate 7 Chipped paint.

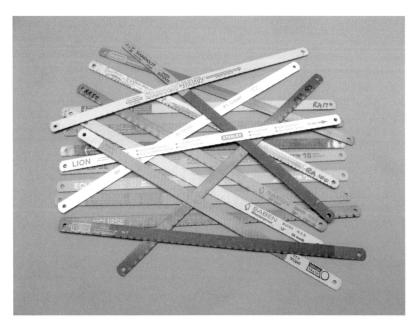

Plate 8 Variety of different hacksaw blades showing that a wide array of colours and colour combinations can be found on them.

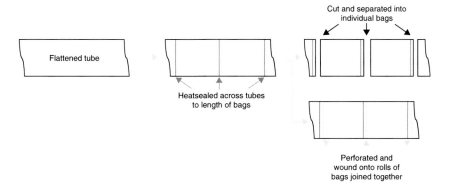

Flattened tube

Heatsealed across tubes to length of bags

Cut and separated into individual bags

Perforated and wound onto rolls of bags joined together

Plate 9 An example of how the flattened tube of film may be transformed into bags by heat sealing, perforating and cutting.

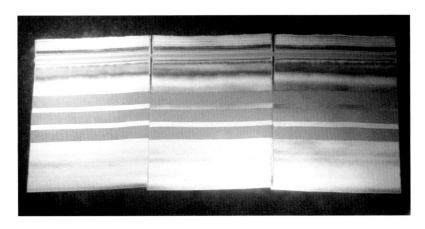

Plate 10 More vivid polarisation colours, using plane polarised light and additional filters.

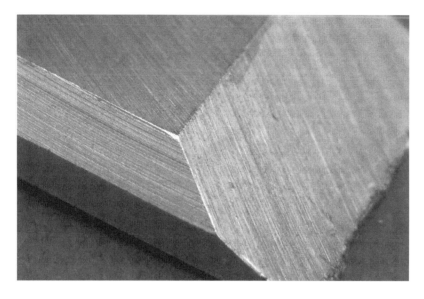

Figure 2.15 Grinding on intersecting faces of a chisel.

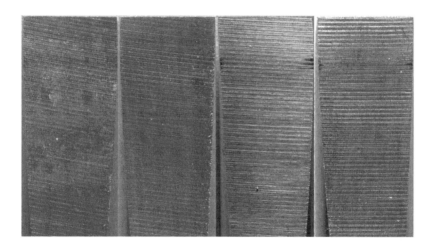

Figure 2.16 Regular grinding detail on simultaneously ground, adjacent blades.

where abrasive particles wear down as a particular groove may stop mid-blade or not continue onto the next.

Re-grinding can also be carried out by hand at home by the owner of a particular tool, to reshape or sharpen it. This could be done using a grinding wheel, which can be used at various angles and leave highly characteristic detail on a tool. A file could also be used for the same purpose, which would leave highly irregular detail as the teeth are pushed and pulled over the tool's

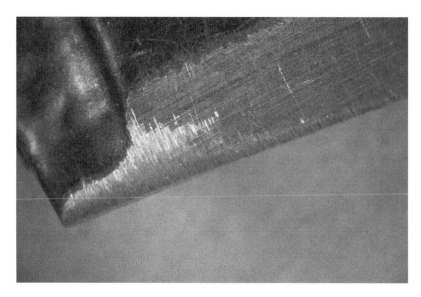

Figure 2.17 A tool blade that has modified detail. The original grinding detail on the bevel is parallel to the tip, with additional grinding at right angles to the tip shown on the left.

surface at various angles. If a sharpening stone were used, this would tend to have a polishing action capable of removing detail from the tool rather than leaving any significant detail of its own. An offender could also use any of these methods in an attempt to modify a tool; for example, by removing or altering detail so that a tool differs from crime scene marks left at earlier scenes, or by significantly reshaping a tool to perform a particular task. An example of a tool with modified detail is shown in Figure 2.17.

Other features that may be seen on the blades of screwdrivers that could be confused with grinding are a series of regular parallel lines pressed across the blade (Figure 2.18). These are generally seen on poorer quality tools that have been produced by a patterned die. Many other screwdriver blades could show the same detail. Tool kits supplied with vehicles often contain screwdrivers with this type of detail.

Tools that are entirely produced from bar stock such as wrecking bars, cold chisels and brick bolsters will have their own integral handle. Other tools will require a handle to be attached or need to be otherwise assembled to form the finished tool. Screwdriver rods may be 'double-winged' where the metal is pinched out at the end of the shaft away from the blade (Figure 2.19), which helps handle attachment. Some tools have a 'tang', which could be an integral extension of the blade as with metal files or knife blades onto which the handle will be attached (Figure 2.20).

Handles are often made out of a variety of plastics or wood, depending on the look and feel required. Injection moulding is often used to produce plastic

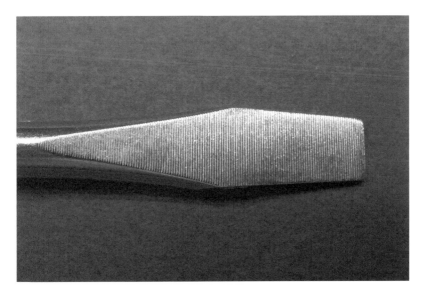

Figure 2.18 Pressed lines on a screwdriver blade.

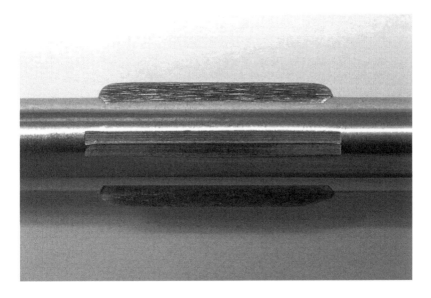

Figure 2.19 Double wings for handle attachment.

handles, which can be done in several steps if a variety different colours and materials are required. The handles can be pressed onto the end of the tool or further fixing such as with glue, rivets and ferrules may be required. Other tools, such as those with forged parts, for example, bolt cutters or shaped

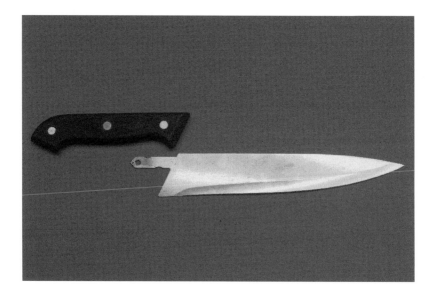

Figure 2.20   A knife blade and tang with handle and rivets.

steel pressings, as with locking pliers, will require assembly and some will
have rubber handles added as well.

Final touches include labelling; for example, etch marking blades such as
wood chisels, printing details onto tools or adding sticky labels for retail
purposes. Some tools such as bolt cutters may have the brand already
forged into the metal, such as Record™. Tools will usually have a quality
control check at some point in their manufacture. This could include a visual
inspection of the quality of the final product and label and whether or not
cracks are present in the metal. Some quality testing involves banging the
work piece on an anvil to see if it sounds dull, as this would indicate a crack
or weakness in the metal, which could cause the tool to fail when used. Tools
that do not meet the standard required are removed from production and
may be scrapped or sold on as seconds. The remaining tools are finished as
appropriate and prepared for sale. Some firms buy in 'unbranded' tools, put
their own markings on and then sell them.

Another point to note is that when tools are produced in batches, they
are often stored together between processes. During storage and also during
processes that involve tools being placed together, such as in a tumbling or
shot-blasting machine, the work pieces can knock together creating small
chips and dents, which may or may not be removed by subsequent processes.
In addition, such practices will lead to consecutively produced pieces, such
as forged bolt cutter blades, becoming mixed up. When they are later
assembled, these pieces would be picked at random and so blades or jaws of
double bladed or jawed items, respectively, are highly unlikely to have been

consecutively made. This mixing up of work pieces, as well as other stages in the manufacturing processes for bolt cutters, is described in more detail in the paper by Butcher and Pugh (1975).

As discussed, in addition to the class features of the tool, manufacturing features that could be useful in a tool mark examination could include any number of the following:

- microscopic irregularities formed during heat treatment and hardening

- shearing and fracture detail or flash

- patterns and defects produced by dies

- surface finish of shot blasted areas

- milling, broaching or grinding detail.

Features present such as those relating to wear and damage can enhance the evidential significance of any matching manufacturing detail between a recovered tool mark and a suspect tool; such features are not produced as part of the manufacturing process, but are randomly acquired throughout the lifetime and use of the tool. Examples of these post-manufacturing modifications are given in the next section.

2.5   Wear, corrosion and damage

Used tools can exhibit highly individual characteristics. The surface of the metal can break down; tips and edges become less sharp and in extreme cases become completely rounded or break off (Figure 2.21). Corrosion could occur and rusty areas could give a pitted or scaly appearance to parts of the tool (Plate 6), or in extreme circumstances the whole tool (Figure 2.22).

Coatings can chip off and flake, leaving irregular outlines on the surface of the tool (Plate 7 and Figure 2.23), which could be shown in a tool mark impression. In addition, a fragment of coating could be recovered from a crime scene, giving the potential for a physical fit of the fragment back to the tool (Figure 2.24) or comparison of any detail retained on the back of the fragment, by virtue of having been applied over grinding detail or similar on the tool's surface (Figure 2.25). Also, if the coating had been applied over grinding or another manufacturing feature, this would leave the detail exposed with the potential to be reproduced in future marks.

Other damage features commonly encountered are scratches, gouges, dents and burrs produced where the tool has contacted a harder surface

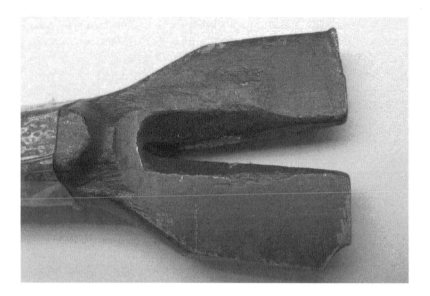

Figure 2.21   Case opener double blade with a broken tip.

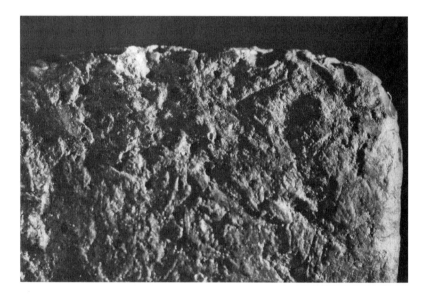

Figure 2.22   A very weathered and corroded tool.

(Figure 2.26). For example, semi-circular notches and burring can be seen in corresponding positions on bolt cutter blades (Figure 2.27), where they have been used to cut through a padlock shackle or other form of hard rod (Figure 2.28); the metal of the blade is compressed and bent around the rod resulting in the shape change and burring.

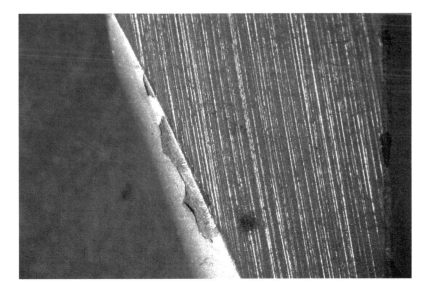

Figure 2.23 Chipped plating.

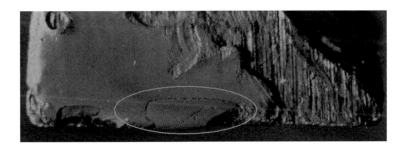

Figure 2.24 Physical fit of a fragment of paint back to a tool.

The damage could be fresh, as revealed by shiny metal with a sharp, cleanly defined appearance (Figure 2.29), or have a weathered appearance, indicating that it is older (Figure 2.30). This could be potentially significant in an examination. For example, if a tool was seized and examined very shortly after an offence, a weathered feature on the tool that did not appear in a clearly defined mark of the same area would suggest that the tool did not make the mark. Conversely, a fresh damage feature could have been made after a tool was used and would not appear in scene marks made by that tool.

Some tools can become completely distorted through use and misuse (Figure 2.31), which could affect which parts of the tool make contact with the substrate and therefore the detail produced by it in a tool mark. Sometimes, distortion can be so extreme it begs the question of whether or not a particular tool could have made the marks at all in its current condition, such as bolt

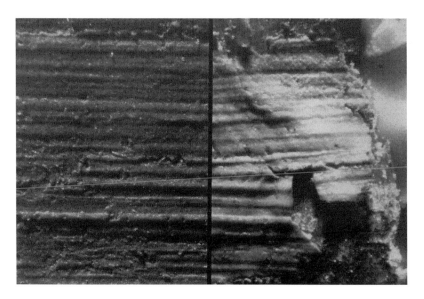

Figure 2.25 Grinding detail on the under surface of a paint fragment (right), chipped off a tool (cast shown left).

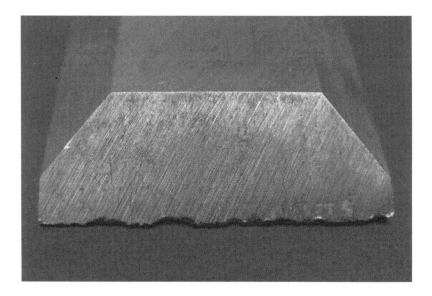

Figure 2.26 Damage to the tip of a chisel.

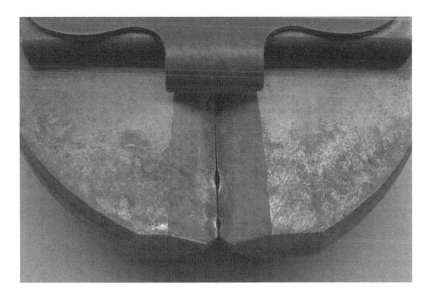

Figure 2.27   Notches on bolt cutter blades.

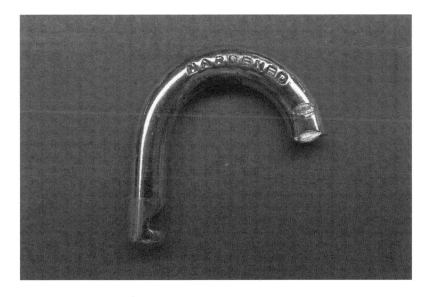

Figure 2.28   A cut padlock shackle.

cutters with jaws so badly set they do not meet properly and could not cut anything. Although, of course, there is the possibility that they may have become damaged making cuts at the scene or subsequently. However, the profile of twisted or misaligned jaws of an operable double bladed cutting tool could be shown in a tool mark.

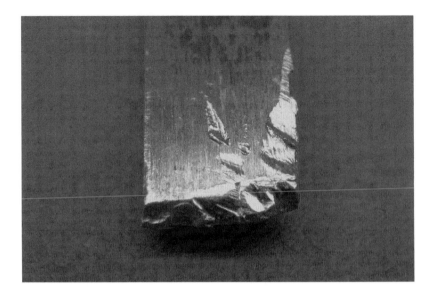

Figure 2.29   Fresh damage.

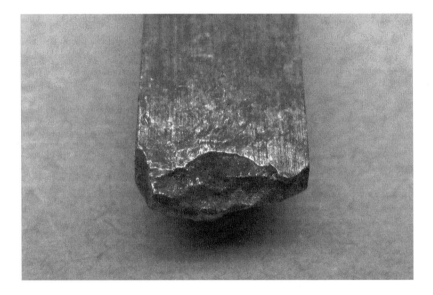

Figure 2.30   Older damage.

It is the combination of the described features, both manufactured and those acquired during use that can make a tool unique in its totality. All tools therefore have the potential to leave identifying characteristics in a tool mark. However, as we shall see, it is often the quality and definition of crime scene marks that are the limiting factors in any comparison.

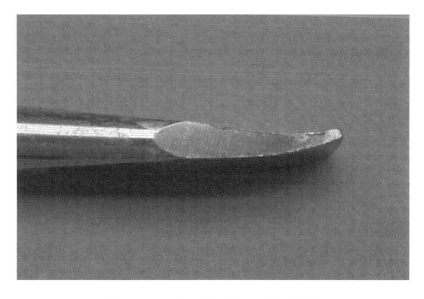

Figure 2.31 Distortion of screwdriver blade.

References

Burd, D.Q. and Gilmore, A.E. (1968) Individual and class characteristics of tools. *Journal of Forensic Sciences*, **13** (3), 390–396.

Butcher, S.J. and Pugh, P.D. (1975) A study of marks made by bolt cutters. *Journal of the Forensic Science Society*, **15** (2), 115–126.

Miller, J. and Beach, G (2005) Toolmarks: Examining the possibility of subclass characteristics. *AFTE Journal*, **37** (4), 296–345.

Monturo, C. (2010) The mechanics of the grinding process. *AFTE Journal*, **42** (3), 267–270.

3
Scene Examination

3.1 Examining and recording the scene

It cannot be said too often or too forcibly that this is one of the most important parts of a tool mark examination. It does not matter how expert the examiner, how good the equipment, if the scene is not properly examined, the correct samples are not taken and a proper record is not made, then, the later laboratory examination can be compromised or rendered useless. While the experienced scene examiner may be able to take short cuts, the general rule must be to proceed carefully, be thorough and do more rather than less.

The following can be no more than guidelines. In the same way that it was difficult to give a short and simple definition of what a tool mark is, so it is difficult to cover all the possible types of scene where marks can occur. The approach taken is to give guidelines and principles for broad types of tool marks, focusing more on how the mark was made than on the type of mark. At the scene there is usually neither the time nor the scope for a detailed examination of the mark itself, so that the main focus must be on the actions that led to the formation of the mark(s) and to the recovery of the mark(s) for later detailed examination at the laboratory. The order of presentation is approximately the same as that which will be used later when discussing the laboratory examination. To avoid too much repetition, each section makes use of information in the previous sections. It should also be appreciated that these guidelines may have to be modified according to the needs of the organization that requires the examination and the requirements of the legal jurisdiction that will be considering the evidence obtained.

The Forensic Examination and Interpretation of Tool Marks, First Edition.
David Baldwin, John Birkett, Owen Facey and Gilleon Rabey.
© 2013 John Wiley & Sons, Ltd. Published 2013 by John Wiley & Sons, Ltd.

3.2   General preliminaries

3.2.1   Verifying the circumstances

Before starting any examination it is worth checking on the previous history of the scene/tool mark, especially for the period of time between when the crime was discovered and the visit of the examiner. Try to find out what the person who discovered the crime did at that time and how the scene was preserved after its discovery. Questions should also be asked about whether a specific mark is relevant; marks can persist for a long time and may have been made previous to the crime being investigated. They may have been made either as a result of a previous attempt (successful or otherwise) to enter the premises at the same point or legitimately by the victim, perhaps having tried to force open a stuck window or door.

It is worth keeping in mind that the first people at the crime scene will not be specialist examiners and may have done things, which seemed perfectly reasonable to them, that will have compromised the mark. Asking questions as early as possible, while matters are still fresh in people's minds, can save much time later. It is far better to ask what can appear to others as silly questions, than to find out later that the mark is irrelevant to the crime.

Another line of enquiry is to check if outbuildings (either at the victim's address or at neighbouring properties) have been entered to obtain tools (such as a garden spade) to gain entry to the main premises. There may be tool marks on these outbuildings that are relevant to the offence. An offender may have brought a 'lightweight' tool with them, but a much more robust tool was required to break in and enter the main premises. The marks on the outbuilding may have been made by the tool that the offender brought and subsequently took away, while the tool used to break into the main premises was left behind.

3.2.2   Recording the scene

Digital cameras are readily available and are the obvious choice to record the general scene details. When scene marks are being recorded it is good practice to include a scale and a label, even in those cases where it is not intended to use the images for later comparison. Review the images before going on to recovering the marks to ensure that they are of acceptable quality and show what was intended.

Written details of these images also need to be made, especially of the location of a mark, so that its position within the general scene may be identified. Again, this could also be recorded in the series of photographs taken at the scene. Also note if the position of the mark places any limitations on how the tool making it could have been used. Photographs taken to show the exact location of the mark in relation to the surroundings may also help to determine this.

In the authors' experience, many police forces in the United Kingdom use scene examination record sheets to give details of the items retrieved and about the examination in general, with added sketches about location, orientation, relative positions of marks, and so on.

3.2.3 Scene to scene linking

Tool marks offer the potential to establish links between offences committed over a period of time, not just on the same day. By recording details about any tool marks recovered, useful intelligence could be gleaned about series of offences where the same tool was used. Scene examiners are unlikely to have suitable equipment to carry out detailed comparisons between marks, but in many cases they could determine a broad category of tool used and obtain a measurement suggesting the size. Even this basic information is better than none, providing that it is capable of being collated. As a minimum, scene examiners could recognise that they have visited several scenes where a screwdriver or other tool was used to gain entry and suggest those as possibly being linked. Most investigating agencies will have crime analysts or similar personnel whose job is to look for emerging patterns; tool marks could be another source of information for them to use, whether by access to crime scene examination reports, entries on crime recording systems or specialised databases. With the information recorded in a searchable format, this intelligence could be available at local, regional or even national level. This is another reason for ensuring that as many marks as possible are recovered from a crime scene. Tools left at a scene by the offender can also be used to search for linked offences (as well as potentially having the offender's DNA or fingerprints on them). More information about using tool marks for intelligence is given in Chapter 4.

3.2.4 Packaging

Items must be properly packaged, not just for transportation to the laboratory, but also for continuity and for secure and safe storage. The items that have been retrieved need to be placed in strong containers that are capable of withstanding rough treatment. Each item needs to be securely packed inside the container so that it cannot suffer damage through poor handling of the package. Items should also be packaged in such a way that any sharp edges or points are protected and cannot cause injury to anyone handling them.

The packaging needs to be secure so that continuity can be maintained and the item cannot be accessed or split out of the packaging once sealed. The packaging should be properly labelled so that the item inside can be identified without opening the package. It is also useful to have on the label the name of the person taking the item, the time and date when the item was taken, the person sealing the item (again with the time and date of sealing) and a reference identifying the investigation/crime that the item relates to. One form of packaging that allows this to be done is the tamper evident bag. The item, with any necessary protection for sharp edges or to prevent damage, is placed into the bag, which has a self-adhesive seal. Once sealed any attempt at reopening the bag reveals a message (such as the word 'VOID') on the seal to show that tampering has taken place. Such bags also usually have a serial number printed on them, usually on the main part of the bag and sometimes on the label area as well. This serial number should be noted on any documentation relating to the item so that subsequent checks could show if the item has been repackaged.

While the packaging requirements outlined above are suitable in most cases, particular care is needed with silicone casts. This is because the full curing process for the cast can take days, even if the cast is hard enough to handle and remove after about 30 minutes. Preferably casts should be packaged into boxes (rather than cylindrical pots) that are large enough for the whole cast to be laid flat. If the cast is distorted in its packing after having been removed from the scene mark, then it will finally harden into the distorted shape. Or, if it has been folded over on itself, the two parts of the cast may set together essentially entombing any detail that may have been present in the relevant area. This potentially may render the cast useless for comparison with a suspect tool. In many cases it will at least make the comparison much harder to undertake and evaluate.

3.3   Forced entry marks—levering

The use of a levering tool to force an entry through a door or a window is potentially the most frequent source of tool marks at scenes of crime (Figure 3.1). Other tools such as hammers and improvised striking tools can be used to force open doors by battering them in. Those, and gripping tools such as wrenches, can be used to damage and remove locks, but these types of attack will be dealt with later in this chapter. Having gained entry to the premises, by whatever means, internal doors, cupboards, drawers, safes, cash boxes and so on may also be forced open, again leading to a source of tool marks.

It is worth looking to see if there are more than just the most obvious marks. What makes a mark obvious is usually the extent and the damage associated with it, which often reduces the quality of the mark. The less obvious marks can have far better detail present in them. As well as checking for marks on the object that has been forced open, the area around the point of attack should be searched. If beading has been forced from a glazed panel as well as marks on the fixed object, the beading may be found on the ground or

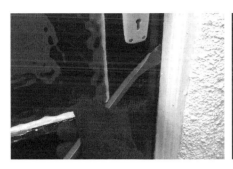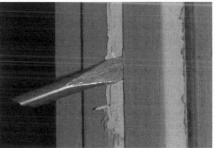

Figure 3.1 Using a levering tool in an attempt to gain access to a door (left) and window (right).

even hidden elsewhere in the vicinity. Likewise, there may be pieces of wood, and so on, that have been broken off during the attack and these may also contain tool marks (Figure 3.2). Forced and damaged door furniture bearing tool marks may also be found on the ground, or still be *in situ* on the door and so can be unscrewed and removed for laboratory examination (Figure 3.3). In addition, consider that if the chisel end of a case opener has been used to lever open a door, the hooked end may have come into contact with the central panel of the door so that area should also be checked (Figure 3.4). If

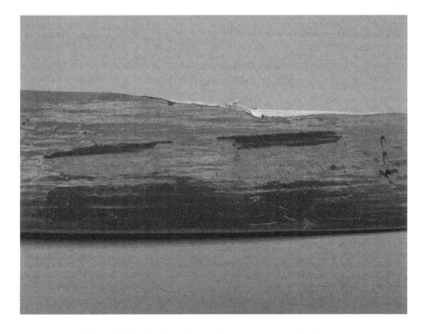

Figure 3.2 Broken piece of wood bearing a tool mark.

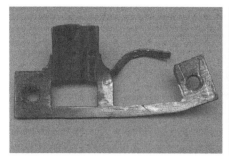
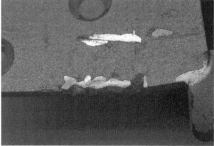

Figure 3.3 Door furniture, as it might be found at a scene (left), may bear limited areas of tool mark, such as those shown (right).

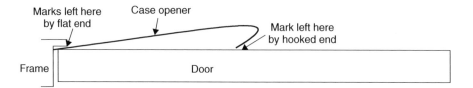

Figure 3.4 Diagram to show marks that may be left by a case opener.

such marks, which can be very shallow, are found, the distance between them and the opening edge should be recorded.

Each time a levering tool is used to force something open there are usually two complementary marks left, which we shall refer to as 'back' and 'tip' marks; for example, one on the door/window and the other on the frame (Figure 3.5). The more obvious are usually the back marks, which are formed at the fulcrum against which the lever presses to create the levering force, and appear as a deep depression on a corner edge of the door/window or frame. The counter mark should be an impression of the tool tip. These may be missed as they may be much shallower and less obvious than the back marks and are mainly on a flat surface. Note the distance between the tip and back mark and also whether this and the orientation give any information on how the lever must have been used.

3.3.1 Recovery of levering marks

The next stage is to consider how any marks that have been found can be recovered for examination in the laboratory. Ideally *all* marks should be recovered, as it is usually impossible at the scene to determine whether any of them contain useful fine, characteristic detail. This can usually only be done in a laboratory using a microscope and suitable lighting (as will be

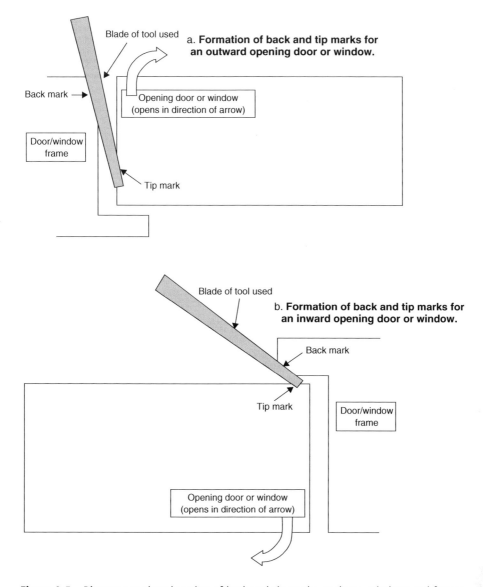

Figure 3.5 Diagrams to show location of back and tip marks on doors, windows and frames.

discussed later in this book). Also, more than one tool may have been used and recovering only a selection of the marks may miss those that have been made by a different tool. By far the best option is to take the item or items bearing the marks for storage or for submission to the laboratory if suspect tools have been retrieved, or to obtain information about the type and size of tool (or tools) that have been used. It is not unknown for complete doors or windows and their frames to be submitted. Submission of the original item also allows the tool mark examiner to search thoroughly in ideal conditions for all the marks that may be present and to recover and record all of them to best effect. If this is not possible then consideration should be given to casting those marks on items that cannot be removed from the scene, using a suitable material, such as those discussed earlier.

Before casting is undertaken, consideration must be given to the possibility of contact trace evidence as the tool must have come in contact with the surface holding the mark. Taking control samples of the surface should be seriously considered. If, for example, the mark is in crushed paint, a sample of the paint from near the mark, but not directly from the mark, should be taken. The only exception to this is when foreign, crushed paint can be seen in the mark and the original mark cannot be removed for laboratory examination. The best approach in this case will depend on the situation. As a general point, the paint used on tools is less likely to provide significant evidence, especially if in a crushed state, than a mark that has identity character present, although paint can be used to provide some corroborating evidence or to eliminate a number of tools from later examination.

One reason sometimes given for not retrieving tool marks, or for taking only one mark when there are several present, is that it takes too long. Often this may be due to not organising the scene examination effectively. Granted there are many other evidential materials to consider at the scene and it does take time for casting materials to set to a point at which they can be removed, but that is usually no more than about 20–30 minutes with modern materials. Even so, if a window or door has been forcibly opened, one good course of action would be to examine that area thoroughly at the start to determine if there are tool marks to be recovered. If these require casting, that process can be started and the casts can be allowed to cure while the rest of the scene is examined, returning to recover the tool mark casts just prior to leaving the venue.

Leaving casting until the end of the scene examination means that there will be 'dead' time while waiting for the casts to set. Under most circumstances the choice of casting material will not be an issue as this will have been determined beforehand, following testing to select suitable moulding compounds, such as those listed in Chapter 1. In some instances, however, the location of the marks to be cast or the ambient conditions may affect the choice. In very cold conditions, such as when casting outdoor marks in winter, a quicker setting variety of casting material may be needed than for the much hotter conditions[1]

---

[1] The notes here generally reflect requirements for temperate climates. For very cold or very hot climates, the initial choice of casting material may well have been influenced by normal ambient conditions for different times of year and there may be different choices made between winter and summer.

that may be encountered indoors or in summer. With two-pack systems the amount of hardener can be varied to take account of the temperature.

Another consideration that is best addressed before going out to the scene is shelf life. There are two different issues here: the effective curing of the material in a reasonable time and 'use-by-date'. The materials should be checked regularly 'at base' to ensure that the casting materials cures to a state in which it can be handled within a recommended time. With a two-pack system, using a fresh batch of hardener will often solve the problem of slow setting and the material can be used. If it still does not cure properly, the material should be thrown away. Even though the material may be past its 'use-by-date', if testing has shown that it still works effectively it can still be used. In either case an audited record should be kept of the testing to show when it was done and that the material was still usable (or show that it failed and was removed from use). Waiting until attending a scene to use the material and finding it does not work is not a viable option.

Downward facing marks can be difficult to cast, as are marks inside restricted areas, such as desk drawers, cash boxes, safes and so on. The main problem, apart from the uncured casting material running out of the mark, is to ensure that the whole mark, including the tip/corners, is cast without trapping air bubbles. One solution is to use a fairly quick setting silicone rubber, which is supplied in a gun, as the material can be applied directly from the nozzle. It is possible to build up the casting material, provided that the detail in the mark is covered evenly first; this will reduce the possibility of the silicone falling out of the mark. If a two-pack system is being used, then a small excess of the hardener can be added, the two components thoroughly mixed, and the resulting thin paste forced into the mark; this needs practice and is not as easy as it is made to sound.

Another possibility is to build up the casting material in the mark by mixing a small quantity of two-pack material or by squeezing a small amount from a gun onto a 'palette', then painting it onto the mark to cover it all in a thin layer before applying the bulk of the casting material on top of that. In each case make sure that there is an excess of silicone rubber to aid later handling. To help getting the casting material into the whole mark, a backing sheet, such as the thin plastic sheets used with fingerprint or footwear mark lifts, or the silanized paper that is used for labelling Isomark™ casts, can be placed onto the back of the casting material as soon as it has been applied and pressing it into the mark.

A different problem is encountered when trying to cast marks in splintered wood. There is no perfect solution to this. One approach is to accept that some of the wood will come away with the cast and to make the cast as bulky as possible, perhaps also including some reinforcing material. Some of the engineering casting materials are designed to be used with recessed, complex shapes and are to be preferred for this type of mark, but they usually take much longer to cure to a state where they can be handled and removed from the mark (sometimes as long as a day) and are better suited to use in the laboratory where they can be left overnight. The casting material is given as long as possible to set, so that it develops its maximum strength, before the attempt is made to remove the cast from the mark. Another approach is to try and use a releasing material, but care must be taken not to obscure any characteristic detail present in the mark. In general, releasing agents do not solve the problem, which is due to the undercut and complex shape that has been left rather than the silicone rubber adhering to the underlying material.

In both the above scenarios another possibility is to use a putty-like moulding compound. While this material is less likely to fall out of a downward facing mark, it should also be remembered that such materials may not take very fine detail. There is a balance to be found here between actually recording some detail of the mark to provide at least some level of evidence and perhaps getting some of the critical fine detail if a high resolution casting material is used, or not recovering the mark at all and having no evidence.

Before the cast has hardened, press a strip of silanized paper onto the exposed surface to aid writing. Such paper is supplied with Isomark™, but another source is the backing sheet from the adhesive films used for lifting footwear marks, which can be cut into suitable size strips for this purpose. When the cast has hardened, use a pen to label it with a reference and also to indicate the orientation of the cast relative to its surroundings. The orientation may need nothing more than two arrows to indicate 'up' and 'inside' for example. For levering marks where there are both tip and back marks, there should be some indication that the pair of casts are linked, such as using sequential numbering. How the casts were marked should be included in the scene record, even in the situation where the scene examiner believes that they will be undertaking the laboratory examination themselves. If the scene examiner has access to a digital camera, a series of photographs could be taken of the casts *in situ* for continuity and to demonstrate how they were orientated at the scene.

In some circumstances, especially when the marks are on a vertical surface (as shown in Figure 3.6) or if the casting material is a mobile liquid, a containing wall or dam could be built round the mark. This is best done with self-adhesive aluminium tape, Blu-Tack™ or plasticine.

Once the casts have been removed from the marks, they should be checked to ensure they have flowed properly into the mark and there are no trapped air bubbles or gaps where the material has started to set early. They should also be checked to see that the casting material has set sufficiently before being removed from the marks. If it has not set sufficiently the surface will be tacky (or even still liquid) and will settle back down losing any detail that may have been present. This can occur either because the casting material has

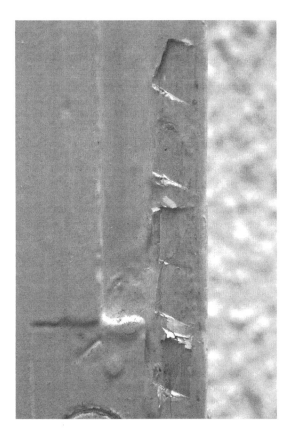

Figure 3.6 Impressed levering marks on a vertical surface, in this case, tip marks made by a screwdriver.

not been properly mixed (usually for two-pack compounds), it has not been left long enough before removal or it is no longer active (old stock). If any of these problems are encountered it is usually possible to cast the mark again.

If original items bearing tool marks have been taken, wherever possible they should also be marked up to show their orientation to the scene and, again, be suitably photographed *in situ* and documented.

3.4   Forced entry marks—other

The previous section dealt with levering marks. As suggested, other tools may be used to force entry to premises or to open doors and other items located inside. The two main methods here are to hit something hard with a hammer, or other improvised striking tool, to break it apart or distort it, such that entry can be gained, or by using a gripping tool such as a wrench or locking pliers to hold and break an object such as a lock. Also included here are some of the methods used to enter or steal motor vehicles using tools.

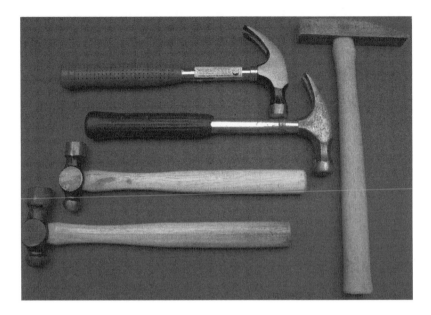

Figure 3.7 Different types of hammer.

3.4.1 Hammer-type attack

When battering an object open, the most likely tool to be used is some form of hammer; these come in many shapes and sizes, from very small cross pein hammers, usually used to drive in small nails or tacks, to sledge hammers used for heavy-duty work (Figure 3.7). However, almost anything could be used to the same effect including heavy tools, such as case openers, bolt cutters and wrenches. Rocks can also be used in this type of situation. The damaged surface, whether it is a door, a cash box or perhaps a vending machine, should be examined carefully for marks as there could be multiple contacts due to repeated blows. Most hammer marks will not show the full shape of the face of the hammerhead, as the blows are usually more glancing (Figure 3.8). Often they will be a combination of striations and partial impressions from the edge of the hammerhead. Careful documentation and recording of these marks *in situ* may be crucial for the laboratory examination, as the location and angle of attack may inform exactly how the tool made contact and help the laboratory examiner to make relevant test marks.

Recovery of these marks is very much in line with the recovery of levering marks. Whenever possible, retrieve the original items bearing the marks intact. Failing that, after checking for contact trace materials, the marks can be cast.

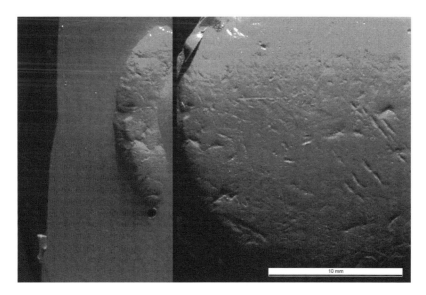

Figure 3.8 Example of a typical glancing hammer mark (cast shown left) and its comparison with a replica cast of a hammer head (right).

3.4.2 Gripping tool attacks

This covers a variety of scenarios where, for example, tools are used to grip, bend and break locks (Figure 3.9) and other door furniture to allow the lock to be compromised, or to grip part of an object to bend and distort it so that access can be gained underneath. Commonly used tools for this type of attack are wrenches, pliers and locking pliers (often colloquially referred to in the United Kingdom as 'mole grips'.). They can also be used to grip padlocks to force them or the fittings away from the object that the padlock is securing.

The common factor in all gripping-type marks is that they should be found in pairs with one jaw making contact with the surface on one side of the object that has been gripped and the other jaw coming into contact with the surface on the other side. It is important to check for marks on both sides, especially if the marks are subsequently going to be cast, rather than retrieving the item bearing the marks. In instances where a door lock has been snapped off there should be grip marks on both sides of the barrel, which will often have been discarded at the scene somewhere. To gain access to the barrel, however, it is normal for the doorplate into which the barrel is set to have been prised, or more likely gripped and pulled upwards, to allow greater access to the lock barrel to give more purchase. The doorplate may still be *in situ*, but heavily distorted, or have broken off and be on the ground nearby. In either case this should be retrieved as well as the lock barrel—one may have better defined

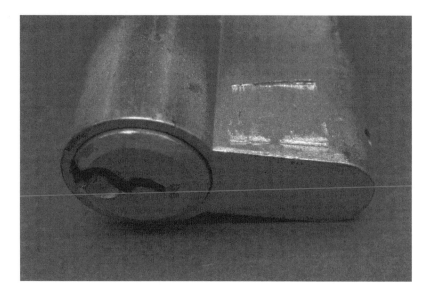

Figure 3.9   A lock barrel with grip marks on it.

detail on it than the other. The door plate may also show shallow levering marks on the under surface where it was initially prised away from the door by a tool such as a screwdriver, again to give better access for the gripping tool.

3.4.3   Motor vehicle entry

The most common methods of illegally entering vehicles by using tools usually involve attacking the locks or door handles. The crudest form is to try to lever out the lock or door handle to gain access to the locking mechanism inside the door. A screwdriver or similar implement is pushed and twisted between the main body panel and lock/handle. This can result in multiple, often overlapping, tool marks on both parts. Ideally the lock/handle should be retrieved for detailed examination at the laboratory. Removing pieces of the body panel bearing marks would be preferable, but is often impracticable, so casting the area is a suitable alternative.

Two other methods employed involve attacking the barrel of the lock by inserting an implement into the keyway. This can be done for both the door locks and the ignition lock. One of these involves pushing a screwdriver or similar tool into the keyway, then twisting it to force the barrel round to operate the lock. The other is the use of a slide hammer. This is a tool normally used to pull dents out of vehicle panels. It has a screw thread at one end (Figure 3.10); this is screwed into the lock keyway (in normal use it would be screwed into the body panel). A heavy weight on the main shaft of the tool is then thrown back and the barrel is pulled out of its housing (or the

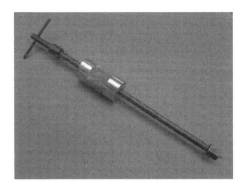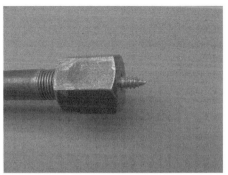

Figure 3.10 A slide hammer (left) with screw thread at one end (right).

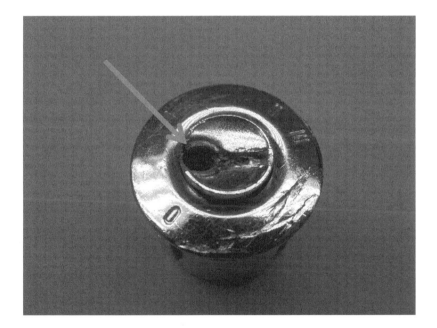

Figure 3.11 Lock barrel with screw hole in keyway.

dented metal panel is pulled outwards). In both cases marks are left inside the keyway by the tool used. Casting these is extremely difficult and so the barrel should be recovered for submission to the laboratory (Figure 3.11).

3.5 Entry by cutting

There are various forms of entry to property or premises, disabling security systems or stealing articles that involve cutting using a variety of different types of tool. The most common tools used for this type of offence are bolt cutters, wire cutters, saws and knives, but secateurs and tree loppers have been used, in addition to more specialised tools such as industrial cable cutters and even 'jaws of life' (hydraulic cutters used by emergency services to free people trapped in motor vehicles).

3.5.1   Padlock removal

A padlock is made up of a body, which contains a locking mechanism, and a shackle, which has an end that can be inserted into the body and then locked. There are many types, ranging across those used for securing sheds, security padlocks for shop shutters, those with large shackles for use with bicycles, those with flexible shackles used to secure otherwise easily removed items and so on. Equally, there are many ways of disabling them and it is unwise to come to a decision too quickly as to which has been used at the scene.

Cutting through the shackle, using a tool such as a pair of bolt cutters, is a fairly quick and quiet method, and therefore commonly used (Figure 3.12). However, it is also possible to break the shackle by levering or using a large wrench on the body, both of which can result in fractured ends that can

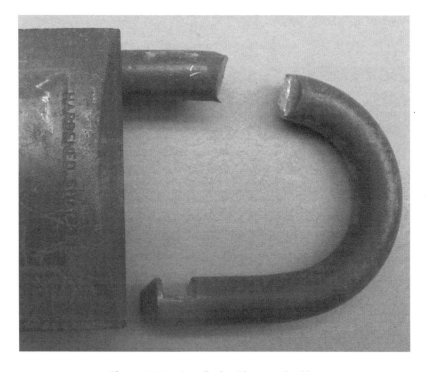

Figure 3.12   A padlock with a cut shackle.

resemble cuts. Always take both the shackle and body for examination if they can be located. It is not always the padlock that has been cut, but instead the staple through which it has been fastened; the lock may be intact, but the staple could be damaged so look for any parts *in situ* and on the ground that may have been cut. If the padlock or fixing appears to be badly distorted and levering is suspected, look for the counter mark, which may be on the object secured by the padlock.

If the padlock is used to secure a chain as a form of security, the chain itself may be easier to cut and any pieces of chain still *in situ*, or pieces of severed chain-link on the ground should be seized.

As a padlock is meant to be portable, the damaged padlock and any pieces of the severed shackle or mountings should be retained and, if necessary, can be sent as a whole to the laboratory. The main effort is in recording the scene and packaging the item(s). Some locks used for securing bicycles have braided metal cables covered with a plastic sheath, sometimes with metal pieces between the cable and the sheath as added protection against cutting. If the bell shapes have been damaged by the cutting tool they may show obvious detail. The braided cable and plastic sheath could also contain useful detail, but this may not be obvious until examined in the laboratory. In some instances there may be detail on the very fine individual wires that make up the cable, which a very experienced examiner may be able to locate and compare with a suspect tool.

3.5.2 Breached security systems

Moving on from cutting padlocks to gain entry to premises or to remove items that have been secured with them, cutting marks can be found in other scenarios where security has been breached. One example involves a physical breach of the security system (such as a fence) to gain entrance and the second involves cutting electrical wire to disable warning security systems or telephones.

Fences around premises may be breached to allow access to either materials in a compound that it surrounds or to gain closer access to premises, which are entered subsequently. One form of fencing, often known as chain-link fencing (as shown in Figure 3.13), is normally made from a hard steel wire, a few millimetres in diameter, coated in plastic to give some protection against the weather. Such wires are often cut using wire cutters or bolt cutters (or similar tools). Because of the small diameter of the wire there is only a small area of cut mark, but there can be more than sufficient detail present for comparison with a tool. So it is important to collect as many ends as possible to enable a good picture of the cutting blade(s) to be obtained. Also, as the core wire is hard steel, the blade(s) may have become damaged during use and the final mark is then noticeably different from the initial mark.

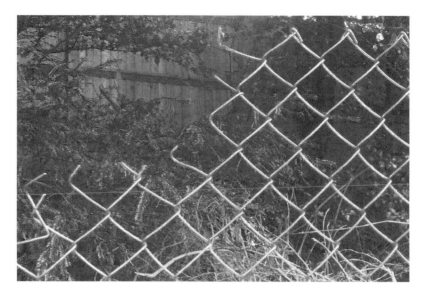

Figure 3.13   A cut chain-link fence.

The scene examiner should search for cut ends of wire still *in situ* on the fence and also pieces of wire that have fallen to the ground. In taking pieces of wire directly from the fence the scene examiner should cut the pieces a few centimetres from the crime cuts. When doing this it is essential that the crime mark cut can be easily distinguished from the scene examiner's cut; for example by suitably labelling the end that is cut by the scene examiner. As a variation on this, the fence may be made from a mesh of small diameter welded steel rods, a material that may also be found with grilles used to protect windows or to make cages. In these circumstances there is often a panel cut out from the mesh. The entire panel should be seized. If possible at least a selection of the remaining mesh should also be taken, again making it clear which are the scene examiner's cuts.

Another type of fencing comprises metal palings pressed from galvanised steel strips (Figure 3.14). These are usually too substantial to be cut by wire cutters and a variety of tools, including bolt cutters and saws, may be used, often along with bending and twisting to effect the final break. It is likely that complete sections of paling have been cut away, but there may also be partial cuts on some of the palings still *in situ*. The examiner should collect any removed pieces, plus complete or partial cuts from the remaining palings (making it obvious which are the examiner's cuts).

Security bars are normally too thick to be cut with standard double-bladed tools (but some specialist cutters generate more pressure and may be used) and saws are the preferred cutting instruments. The removed bars can be packaged for later laboratory examination and the cut ends of the pieces that

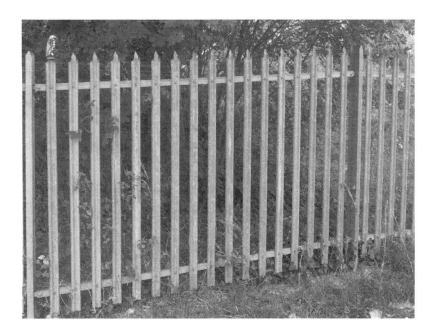

Figure 3.14   A fence comprising galvanised metal palings.

are still in place can be cut off by the examiner for submission. A different technique is to use a vehicle to either pull out the bars or force them in. When used on the shutters used to protect shop fronts this is known as 'ram raiding' in the United Kingdom. This type of attack rarely leaves usable tool marks and it is better to concentrate on contact trace evidence.

Electrical 'wires' can range in size from the very fine individual telephone wires to heavy duty, high-voltage cables. The latter are more usually cut in order to steal the cable for the value of the metal rather than for bypassing security. Alarm and telephone cables on the outside of premises may be cut to disable security; this can include cutting larger telephone cables running into industrial premises. Finding the location of the cut wire may be an issue in this last case. The type of tools used can range from wire cutters, bolt cutters, pruning tools and specialist cutters to knives and saws. In some instances the wires may have been pulled apart by hand. For each 'cut' in the wire there will two ends that should be recovered; these could be still *in situ* or on the ground nearby (unless the intention was to steal the cable). They should be recovered as for cut fencing and similar wires.

The small diameter of most electrical wire, especially the inner metal core, means that it is very difficult, but not impossible, to obtain useful results concerning the tool from a laboratory examination. This is especially true for telephone wires, where the inner conductor is usually a thin metallic film on a plastic core. It is, however, often possible to determine the class of tool used to cut these wires, which may be of assistance in the case. A thorough microscopic examination in the laboratory may show the presence of detail on the plastic sheathing or even on some of the individual metal wires forming the core (in the same way as on braided bicycle chains mentioned earlier). Every case needs to be assessed in relation to the needs of the investigation, but where cut wires are involved questions need to be asked about what these needs are and what the investigating officer's expectations are concerning the laboratory examination to be undertaken. Although expectations may be low, without a detailed examination of the cut wires it is not possible to determine exactly what type of tool has been used or if there is any useful detail on the cut ends.

3.6   Theft of metal

Theft of metal has already been alluded to with respect to heavy duty, electrical cable. Other types include theft of lead or lead sheet from the roofs of buildings, theft of copper piping and associated fittings (including boilers and radiators) and the theft of lightning conductor strips together with any other accessible metal items.

When large power cables are targeted, these can be centimetres in diameter and have a woven steel sheath under the insulation to provide protection to the inner multi-strand copper core. The main problem in collecting can be in physically cutting the cable to sample it, while preserving the relationship of the individual strands of wire and sheathing. A specialist cable-cutting tool, if the victim has access to one, can be one solution. Smaller diameter, or more loosely packed, cables can be more prone to displacement of the individual strands, so binding them together with tape before sampling is advisable so long as this is documented to show it was part of the sampling process and not a feature of the original cable.

Lead (and sometimes copper) sheet is used as an external building material. Removal techniques include using case openers, claw hammers or other levering tools to prise the material from its fixing. All of these potentially leave marks in the underlying material, which can be recovered by casting. If some of the metal is still present at the scene either *in situ* or lying around, this could also be checked for evidence of any tool marks. These may include gripping marks where pliers or similar tools have been used to pull away the lead. In most instances lead sheet is torn rather than cut during the theft, cut marks often being part of the original process when the lead was fitted to the roof. Check as far as possible that the marks found are related to the crime and not part of the original building process, which includes cutting the sheet to size.

Copper piping and other fittings are often stolen from buildings. The piping and fittings can be levered from their fixings and this leaves marks in the underlying building material. If these marks cannot be removed they will need to be cast. In some cases pipe cutters or saws are used to cut the copper pipe, although in many cases the piping may simply be bent to break it. In these cases the potentially cut ends should be taken for laboratory examination to either compare with tools from a suspect or to identify what type of implement (if any) has been used.

A recent development in criminal activity is the theft of catalytic converters from vehicles; these are normally part of the external exhaust system. For this, the exhaust system is cut on either side of the catalytic converter and the two remaining cut ends should be taken for examination. The types of tool used for this type of theft include saws, grinding discs (angle grinders), pipe cutters designed for this purpose with several cutting discs arranged on a chain that fits round the exhaust and even heavy duty hydraulic cutters, each of which leave their own form of marks.

Where theft of metal is concerned, it is the weight of the metal that is important to the thief. Where power cables are concerned the outer sheathing may be stripped off by the offenders. This is often done by burning, but in some cases the sheathing may be stripped off using commercial machinery. The metal may also be cut into pieces that are easier to handle, perhaps using an industrial guillotine or other specialist cutter. In such cases, it may be possible to link the machinery back to relevant materials that have been recovered. Where possible the machinery should also be recovered. However, if the machinery is not particularly portable, such as a powered guillotine, then a visit to the workshop where it is situated may be in order. This will be described in more detail in the next section.

3.7   Examination of machines

There are occasions when large pieces of equipment are suspected of having been used in a crime. Some of these have been referred to earlier in this chapter (e.g. cable stripping machinery and industrial guillotines). Others can arise where an illicit drugs factory has been discovered. Equipment found there could include a tablet press or moulds used for pressing drugs into blocks. Similarly with fake currency, where stamping presses are used for coins and printing presses for banknotes. The equipment for making fake credit and similar cards usually comprises relatively small machines that can be seized intact, but others can be difficult to move and are better examined at the scene.

Where it is not possible to bring the relevant part of a machine for laboratory examination it will be necessary to examine the machine *in situ*. These are always potentially difficult examinations as it is necessary to ensure that someone who knows how to operate the machine is present. The operator should ensure that the machine is safe to use before any attempt is made to use it to produce test marks. Also it is necessary to ensure that power to operate the machine is available before going to the scene. Pre-plan the visit with care and make provision for contingency time; it always takes longer than expected. Make sure that there is not only enough material to prepare the required control items but also sufficient to undertake a few trial runs beforehand. Take at least two sets of controls items, so that it is possible to estimate how variable the marks are. It is important to take sufficient control items for the later examination, as it will be difficult and costly to arrange a return visit.

3.8 Pathology samples

There are two main situations where tool marks may be recovered from a victim's body (alive or dead). In cases involving assault with an implement of some kind, including when a victim has been punched by someone wearing rings or a knuckleduster, the mark will nearly always be some form of bruising. Under these circumstances the victim may have died, but more often will still be alive. Such marks are best photographed by an experienced photographer.

There are two main points of concern. The first is that because the human body does not have any really flat surfaces, flexible tape scales are used to provide a scale. For later marks' comparisons a rigid scale needs to be included as well, even if only to be sure of the scale of the reproduced image used for the comparisons. This requirement is not optional but a necessity. The second point is that some marks are better imaged using near-infrared or ultraviolet light, which requires specialised equipment. These points need to be discussed before having the photographs taken. Another point is that the mark(s) can develop over a period of time—say, a few days—and photographs taken at a later date can prove useful; even if the victim has died, the bruising may show more clearly as it can develop *post mortem*.

In the situation where the person is dead, tool marks are likely to fall into several categories—stab marks (Figure 3.15), impacts from tools such as hammers and axes (Figure 3.16) and marks left by cutting up a body. Normally the samples of such marks will be taken by a pathologist. This requires good

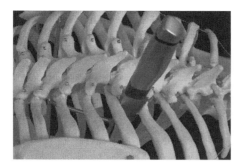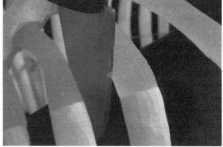

Figure 3.15 Insertion of a knife between the ribs from the back (left) and front (right) during a stabbing, could leave cut marks in the bone and/or cartilage.

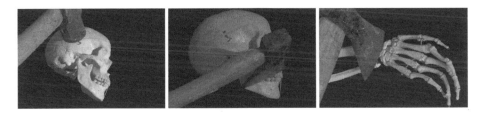

Figure 3.16 How a hammer or an axe might be used on different parts of the body.

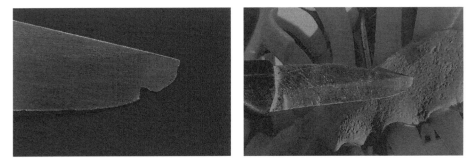

Figure 3.17 How a characteristic knife blade could leave a very shallow mark in bone, capable of providing a specific link to the correct knife.

liaison, so that both the pathologist and the marks' examiner understand the limitations imposed on the pathologist and the possibilities arising from the marks' examination. In particular, there is a need to emphasise that it is not size that is important but the quality of the mark. A mark in bone, no more than a millimetre wide and deep (or even less), say from the tip of a knife, can be used to identify the tool making the mark (Figure 3.17). It should also be remembered that, as with all other tool marks, there may be several different marks on a section of bone and whenever possible they should all be recovered. The potential of recovering marks from bones and comparing them with a suspect tool was recognised in a paper originally published by Thomas and Gallent (1947) and reprinted in the *AFTE Journal* of Spring 2007. The present authors would stress, however, that procedures have advanced since then and they do not agree with making test marks in another body!

Ideally the victim's injuries will be photographed as part of the normal post-mortem procedure and these should clearly show the location and relative orientations of any marks, especially on severed bones. This is particularly important where both the radius and ulna or tibia and fibula have been cut, as they could allow the marks' examiner to determine whether the marks relate to both bones being cut at the same time, or if they have been cut separately

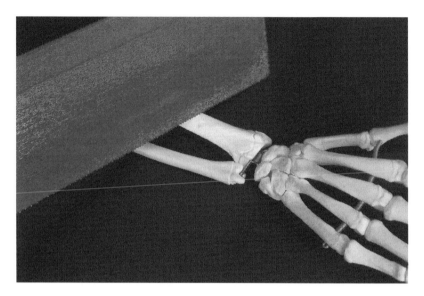

Figure 3.18   How a saw could cut simultaneously through two bones, in this case the radius and ulna of the arm.

(Figure 3.18). This applies not only to marks where the bones have been severed, but also for any partial cuts. Samples of bones bearing the marks should be taken whenever possible, but this must be done with due respect and in accordance with any legislation relating to human body tissue.[2]

Where bones have been cut through, there is a need to identify the crime cut and distinguish it from the pathologist's cut. This can be done in various ways and must be fully documented for future reference so that it is obvious to the marks' examiner that all cuts/marks made by the pathologist can be accounted for. The pathologist will need to remove most of the soft tissue surrounding the bone but they need to be aware that it should be done in a way that does not produce new marks on the bone.

In very exceptional circumstances, often involving torture, the victim may still be alive but have potential tool marks on parts of the body; these can include toes or fingers being cut off, teeth being forcibly extracted or impacts on the skull where the skin has been broken exposing the bone underneath. Unless there is a good medical reason, it is obvious that taking relevant pieces of bone will not be an option here (although extracted teeth and possibly cut off appendages may be an option if taken with appropriate authorisation and consent of the victim or other responsible person). Medical advice may be necessary, but if the marks are exposed and the area can be kept clean, dry and sterile, casting may be possible.

---

[2] In the UK this currently falls under the *Human Tissue Act* (Government Legislation, 2004).

Submissions to the laboratory should include not only the casts and pieces of bone, but also copies of the post-mortem photographs showing the injuries and a copy of the pathologist's report.

This is an awkward area for liaison, as it is unlikely that the pathologist and marks' examiner will be in frequent contact. Wherever possible, professional links should be developed through attending joint meetings or by arranging meetings for practitioners in the area. Without an awareness of what is practicable in general, expectations are built around high-profile cases that have produced exceptional results. When these are not achieved for the more typical cases, then there is a tendency not to repeat the examination, even though useful results could have been obtained. Another aspect of the problem is that, unless these professional links have been developed, it is unlikely that either the investigating officer or the pathologist will contact a marks' examiner before the sample is taken, which may cause problems with any later marks' examination.

3.9 Collecting suspect tools

When it is necessary to collect suspect tools, it is better to collect all the tools that could have possibly made the mark of interest. Normally these will be seized in connection with the suspect(s), but some may also be found at the scene of crime. Remember that some types of saw have removable blades and any discarded blades should also be seized, as should pieces of broken blade that may have been used. Once seized, the tools should be suitably packaged for continuity and to allow for possible subsequent examination for contact trace materials, including DNA, or fingerprints. If the protocol of the submitting authority allows for early swabbing for DNA or examination for fingerprints, to establish a potential link between suspect and tool (for example, if the tool is found in the back of van), before submission to the laboratory, this needs to be documented as it may preclude subsequent examination of those tools for other contact traces.

The tools should also be suitably packaged to prevent, or at least limit, any subsequent damage (Figure 3.19). The two ways of packaging shown are using a weapon tube that completely encloses the tool (upper) and just covering the tip with a small plastic tube taped in place (lower). Although the weapon tube can be sealed with tape and a label attached without further packaging, the use of a tube over the end of the blade would require further packaging in a sealed bag, to retain any trace material that may be further up the shaft. Another suitable form of packaging a tool would be to tie it into a strong cardboard box and either seal that shut or place the box in a sealable bag.

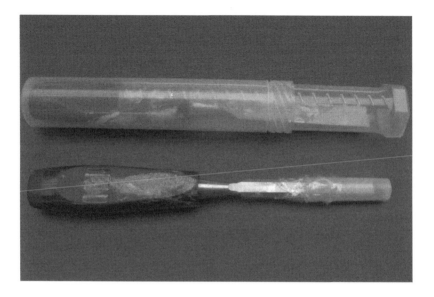

Figure 3.19   Examples of how tools may be packaged to protect the working end.

This is another example of where it is easier to review the items away from the scene. It also allows for the possibility that the later laboratory examination indicates a specific tool that had not been considered during the initial scene examination. In cases where large numbers of tools have been seized, a sensible course of action could be for the marks to be submitted to the laboratory, where a detailed examination is carried out to gather information about the most relevant tools to be submitted for comparison. Indeed, the tool mark examiner should consider going to a suitable location to screen through all the tools that have been seized, rather than just providing information and allowing a third party to select the relevant tools. In this way the examiner has looked at all the tools and can select all potentially suitable tools and comment that the others were all of the wrong type to have made the marks.

When tools are submitted to the laboratory, it may seem sensible to provide only the tool(s) from a suspect who is not admitting the offence and for the police to retain any tool(s) from a suspect who has admitted involvement or tools recovered from the scene. This can be a false economy. If two very similar tools were found on different suspects and only that from the person who is denying involvement is submitted, the scientist may spend a long time trying to positively eliminate (or link) that tool. However, if the second tool had also been submitted, it may be easily linked to the marks, precluding the needed for a detailed comparison of the first tool (saving time and money).

In addition to tools recovered from the scene of crime, the possibility of a tool having been damaged at the scene should also be considered. It is not unknown for a tool tip to be broken off during forcible entry and it could be found on the ground or even embedded in the door furniture. As will be discussed in Chapter 8, a tool tip could potentially be linked back to the tool from which it came, but there is also the possibility that the tip itself (as well as tools found at the scene) could be compared with marks recovered from earlier offences to provide links between them.

References

Government Legislation/Act of Parliament (2004) *Human Tissue Act*, http://www .legislation.gov.uk/ukpga/2004/30/contents (accessed October 2012).

Thomas, F. and Gallent, G. (1947) Homicide by blows dealt to the head by means of an axe and identification of the weapon. *International Criminal Review*, 10 August to September 1947. Reprinted (2007) in *AFTE Journal*, **39** (2), Spring, 88–94.

4
Initial Laboratory Examination

4.1 General preliminaries

4.1.1 Receiving items

Without sufficient information regarding the state of affairs surrounding the event in question, it is not always possible to undertake a meaningful marks' examination. This is a problem that is often not recognised by either the laboratory administration or the investigating officer. Details concerning the events relating to the crime together with the investigating officer's needs and expectations are both required to carry out a tool mark investigation effectively. Both groups of people are more used to the situation where a sample is submitted to the laboratory, say for a simple drug or DNA analysis, the scientist doing whatever is needed and then returning an answer. For these cases, a simple reception area is all that is needed, where the case samples can be delivered, logged in and securely stored. The samples will normally be submitted with a pro forma that contains sufficient information to allow the scientist to carry out the examination. There is often considerable resistance from both parties to any change to this system.

There are a number of reasons why the pro forma approach does not work for tool marks. One is that the investigating officer may not have dealt with many tool mark cases; in fact the one being submitted could well be the first. They can be unaware of the problems involved in using tool mark evidence. The other is that after the initial questions, the secondary questions are very dependent on the answers first received. For example, it is necessary to confirm that the questioned tool can be connected to the suspect at the

The Forensic Examination and Interpretation of Tool Marks, First Edition.
David Baldwin, John Birkett, Owen Facey and Gilleon Rabey.
© 2013 John Wiley & Sons, Ltd. Published 2013 by John Wiley & Sons, Ltd.

time of the crime. If the tool was recovered in the suspect's possession a day or more after the crime was committed, then it will be necessary to show that no one could have 'borrowed' it to commit the crime. Unless the officer has covered this aspect of the investigation there is little point in undertaking the tool mark examination.

If there has been a delay of more than a day it is also necessary to check whether the tool could have been used after the crime. If the suspect has a legitimate trade where the tool could have been used, the working edge profile may have changed and this needs to be considered.

There are further questions to be asked about whether the tool needs to be examined for fingerprints, DNA or contact trace evidence. If this is the situation, it is nearly always better to have these examinations carried out before the tool mark examination.

There are also questions concerning the needs and expectations of the investigating officer in regards to the examination. Is a strong result or identification required, or will matching class features be sufficient? Tool mark examinations can take a long time to complete, so is there a date when the results (statement) must be with the investigating officer? It is sensible to use this discussion to get a genuine contact point (e.g. telephone number, email address), rather than having to go through a call centre, as the early examination can often indicate that the needs and expectations as discussed cannot be met and need to be modified.

This information is best gathered at the laboratory by the tool marks' practitioner who will be working on the case, from the submitting officer, who should also be the investigating officer. It needs suitable surroundings, a table and chairs in a quiet area at least. It does not have to take a long time; with experience 15 minutes should be sufficient. The discussion must be recorded and the notes taken during the discussion may be sufficient. Once in place and working, the benefits become apparent but the problem is to get the system in place to start with.

4.1.2   Planning the examination

Examining tool marks is not a conveyor belt process where the items start at one end, go through a standard set of processes and an answer appears at the other end. Therefore, planning is needed if the best results are to be obtained in an acceptable time. Firstly, read the paperwork submitted with the case and review the notes taken during the discussion with the submitting officer. From these make some preliminary decisions concerning what examinations will be required and roughly how long they may take. Here it is necessary to distinguish between working time and elapsed time. Working time is the time spent in undertaking active work on the case. Elapsed time is the amount of time between the case coming in for examination and the report leaving.

For many types of forensic science case there is little difference between the two, but for tool mark examinations, where there can be periods of inactivity while waiting for other parts of the examination to develop, there can be significant differences. Make sure that there is sufficient elapsed time for the examination to meet its deadline.

The type of considerations to be taken into account are availability of equipment and key personnel, periods when it will be necessary to wait for results and known interruptions that will take the examiner away from the laboratory bench. Because there are gaps between the working time periods, availability of equipment becomes important, as a tool mark examiner will need to be working on more than one case to make effective use of their time. However, it is poor practice, if for no other reason than possible cross contamination, to have two sets of case items open on the same bench. Similar considerations apply to use of major equipment, such as a tool mark comparator, as well as allowing for its use by other people.

A further consideration is the order in which the items should be examined. Theoretically, it is best to examine the questioned marks first, so that an unbiased opinion can be formed concerning the class features and any identity characteristics of the tool that made them. Practically, if there are many questioned marks it can be more sensible to examine the tool first and determine if any of the marks can be eliminated because they have different features. Also, if contact trace evidence is part of the examination, the tools and the marks should at least be examined on separate benches if not in separate rooms.

In complex cases there may be more than one scientist involved, so that it will be necessary to liaise with them to determine if any of the items need to be examined by more than one scientist. If multiple examinations are required, it is important to establish priorities and agree on how they are to be conducted. Approximate times also need to be established for when the examinations are likely to take place so that the total case examination can be carried out effectively.

If there is a potential need for assistance from other people, such as professional photographers, scanning electron microscopists or similar, then some time must be allowed for their work. This can be amended as the examination progresses and it becomes clearer what will be needed. In addition, allowance needs to be made for planned and unplanned interruptions. Planned interruptions will be in the examiners office diary but unplanned interruptions can only be estimated from experience. Such matters as court attendance, answering telephone inquiries, gathering information on newly submitted cases and so on do take an appreciable time and can account for around 20% of the elapsed time for an examination.

4.1.3   Preparing for the examination

Good preparation and organisation can be key to a timely examination. By ensuring that all of the equipment that one may need, as described in Chapter 1, is available and ready for use nearby, the examiner will avoid unnecessary trips to and fro when the examination has started. The working area needs to be prepared for use. Wiping down the working area using a damp, clean and disposable cloth, with sweeping motions off the edge will help to ensure that any particulate matter has been removed and fresh brown paper or other cover can be laid down.

4.1.4   Collecting the items

Even in those cases where the tool mark examiner has met the submitting officer, the normal practice is to place the items in a secure store until they can be taken into the laboratory area for examination. When collecting the items for examination, check the items against the file records to ensure that they are all present. Make a record of the transfer in the file, signing and dating it. If the transfer is from a colleague, additionally make a note on whether the item packages are sealed and get your colleague to sign and date your transfer record.

4.1.5   Decontamination of item packaging

A serious and perennial concern for forensic science laboratories is one of contamination. As search, recovery and analytical techniques become more sophisticated, smaller and smaller amounts of material can be used to provide a link between crime scenes and items. It is very easy to transfer small amounts of material from the outer packaging of the item to the examination area accidentally. It is advisable to wipe down the outer packaging before placing an item on the examination bench.

4.1.6   Operating procedures

It has taken quite a time to reach this point, but the items have not yet been opened for the initial examination. The question of whether all the preceding is necessary is a natural one to ask. How this is answered depends on both the jurisdiction and the organisations that have commissioned the examination. The underlying problem is that there are competing demands between comprehensive, accurate and dependable results against cost effectiveness coupled with timeliness. How these are resolved depends on the requirements of the various organisations. To achieve dependable results most laboratory administrations will have written standard procedures and these are often the basis for accreditation of the laboratory by an outside organisation for the laboratory's work.

Most forensic science laboratories are multidisciplinary and the operating procedures reflect this; some laboratories require the examiner to change all their outer clothing for laboratory clothing to minimize contamination. Other laboratories undertake examinations that are less susceptible to cross contamination and have a more relaxed approach. It is therefore important to read the operating procedures thoroughly and to follow them. If the reasons for a procedure are not clear then the examiner should ask for clarification. Equally, if some point seems to have been missed then this also needs to be clarified. If the matter cannot be satisfactorily clarified then the procedure should be rewritten. Broadly speaking, all the points covered above should appear somewhere within the given procedures.

The standard procedures encapsulate the laboratory's response to the need for dependable results given the time constraints and costs. Of necessity, they do not cover all eventualities and the examiner may need to extend or modify a given procedure for a particular examination. In both situations, detailed notes are required, preferably including a reference to the published work on which the changes are based. It must be recognised that the examiner is ultimately the person responsible for the examination and so must be prepared to be held accountable for the results obtained.

4.1.7 Recording and opening the packaging

Two things need to be recorded, the labelling on the packaging and the state of security of the package. The labelling is most easily recorded using a digital camera, the images being printed for inclusion in the examination file. A written record is possible but can be time consuming. The packaging needs to be examined to determine whether it was possible for contaminants to have entered and to verify the security of the item. If it is clear that the package has been opened and resealed at some earlier time, check the labelling to find out if there is a record of this. If not, check with the investigating officer to find out if they know why the package needed to be opened and how the item was handled while the package was open.

As the condition of the package sealing may be important to the court, it is sensible to open the package in a way to leave the original sealing intact. From a practical point of view, it is also sensible to remember that the package is going to have to be resealed and to open it in a way to make the resealing as easy as possible. In some instances, it will not be practical to open the packaging so that it can be re-used and resealed after the examination. Under these circumstances the examiner should retain the original packaging and labelling so that it can be returned with the repackaged item, recording that this has been done. The protocol of some submitting authorities (or for certain types of case) may insist that once the packaging has been opened the item and original packaging must be placed into new sealed packaging after the examination. Any repackaging should be properly documented.

4.1.8   Description of the item

Remove the item from the packaging, taking due consideration of other examinations that may be required and taking suitable precautions, and check that it matches the description given in the documentation and labelling. Make a record of the item; include a scale and a label with the item reference, whether this is done by digital photography, photocopier or some other method.

4.1.9   Examination of the item

Up to this point the general procedure will be the same for whatever item has been submitted. In what follows, the procedure depends on the type of item and the information required from the examination. This involves a change in view point from that taken for scene examination, where the type of scene was the important consideration, to one where the type of mark is the important consideration.

This will be the first time that the item has been examined under laboratory conditions, even if the examiner collected the items. It is necessary to get rid of any preconceived ideas regarding the marks, for example that they are going to be impressed or sliding marks, and examine the item objectively to determine what can be inferred from the mark and the best approach to the subsequent course of examination.

Another point to be borne in mind is that it may be possible at this initial stage of the examination to eliminate the mark from being of use to the investigation. Knowing that the mark/tool combination can be eliminated is just as important to the investigating officer as knowing that there is some link between them.

Use the maximum overhead lighting available and also use a secondary, directional light to illuminate the individual marks. A hand lens may be of use at this stage. If there are a number of marks on the same item, record their positions and label them for future reference. For cut marks also note and record individual cut surfaces in each mark.

4.2   Mainly impressed marks

This section essentially covers some types of levering marks, impact marks and gripping marks, which can all be dealt with in similar ways.

A microscopic examination at around $\times 10$ will reveal any characteristic detail present, especially when aided by oblique illumination from a secondary source. If a long-arm microscope is being used, the examination can sometimes be made easier where small items are concerned by positioning the microscope head over the edge of the workbench and manipulating the item by hand to bring features of interest into view.

The first point to note is the shape of the mark, as this can help to determine the general type of tool that has been used. Has it been made by a levering tool (such as a screwdriver or case opener), is it an impact mark (such as that left by a hammer) or is it a gripping mark (such as from locking pliers, a wrench or a vice)? Also, for each item note how many marks are present.

4.2.1 Levering marks

For levering tools, if both edges are present in the mark, note if the blade is parallel sided or if it tapers or widens towards the tip. For example, many (but not all) case openers and chisels have parallel sides, whereas screwdrivers usually taper or widen towards the tip (Figure 4.1). Also, check to see if the width of the blade can be measured at a defined place such as the tip or where the edges of the blade change direction. If the forked end of a case opener (or claw hammer) has been used, there will usually be marks made by both prongs and additional information can be gained by checking the shapes and measurements for both as well as the spacing between them (Figure 4.2).

Attention should be paid to any corner marks left by the tool; is the corner sharply defined or has it become rounded due to wear? Is there

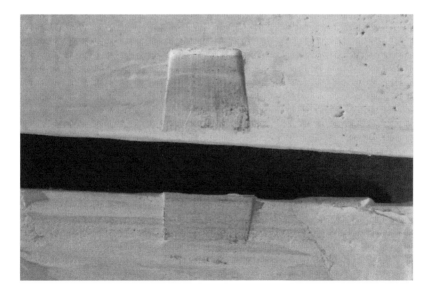

Figure 4.1 Screwdriver tip (top) and back (bottom) marks in painted wood. The top mark shows that the screwdriver tapers towards the tip.

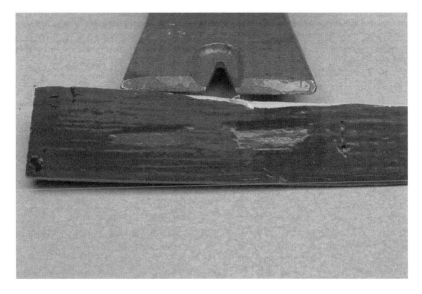

Figure 4.2 A typical impressed mark made by two prongs of a case opener. Obviously, any contact traces should have been recovered prior to bringing the tool and mark together, also care should be taken not to create any further marks on the scene item.

any evidence of significant damage, such as a missing (irregular) corner or burring (Figure 4.3)? Examine the edges of the mark to determine if there is any evidence to suggest that either the tip of the tool (or edges of a tool if something like a wood chisel has been used) is bevelled or if there are any characteristic features left by wear damage to the tool.

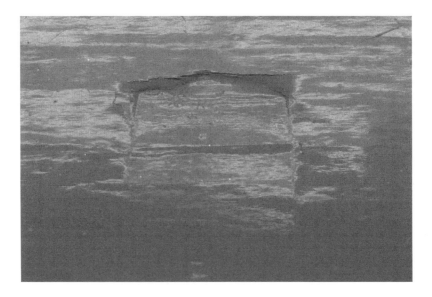

Figure 4.3 A levering mark made by a bladed tool with a characteristic tip profile.

Caution should be exercised in determining if a tool is bevelled or not. Bevelling may not be obvious if there is a very shallow mark where only the main body of the blade has made contact. There can also be some apparent bevelling when an unbevelled blade has slipped and dug into the surface at an angle during use to leave striations and shapes similar to that expected for a bevel.

Examine the nominally flat surfaces present in the mark; are there any potentially characteristic features present? Such features could include ridges, pits, chipped paint or plating and so on, as well as possible grinding detail. At this stage of the examination, unless the features are especially clear, it is unwise to assign them specifically to damage on the tool face. Without further information it can be difficult to differentiate between damage and other possible features that are due to some other process. If there is any clear grinding or pressed detail on the surface of the blade responsible for the mark, the direction should be noted.

Although the majority of the mark may be a clear impression, it is worth checking to see if there is any sliding detail present. If there is, it is normally towards the point at which the tip or edge of the tool has come to rest. At this stage it is best just to note that striations are present; if the striae are curved and parallel, then it is more likely that they are sliding marks than impressed grinding detail.

If there are other marks available, these should also be checked to see what detail they contain. It should not be assumed that all marks, even those of similar size and type, have been made by the same tool. Any dimensions that are present, for example the width of the blade tip or the separation of a forked end, should be estimated for each of them wherever possible. A ruler or a calliper gauge measuring to the nearest millimetre can be used for this purpose. When potentially characteristic features are present in several marks, they should be checked against each other to see if they appear to be reproducible and therefore a reliable characteristic of the tool.

4.2.2 Impact marks

For impact marks note the overall shape (Figure 4.4). This will often not include the whole face of the tool used, but will often just be one edge. Is it straight or rounded? Is there a well-defined bevelled edge present? Is the edge rounded and worn? Can any dimensions be taken, for example the diameter or width of the hammer head (depending on shape)? Is there any potentially characteristic detail present? Remember that tool marks can look different depending on what substrate they have been made in, as shown by the hammer mark made in painted hardboard in Figure 4.5.

4.2.3 Gripping marks

For gripping marks, there should be two related impressions on either side of the object that has been gripped and these could show differences in general

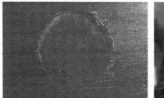 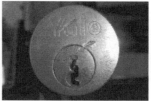 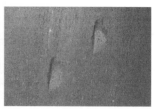

Figure 4.4   An impression from the full face of a hammer head (left), a partial hammer mark (middle) and an impact mark from the head of a golf club (right).

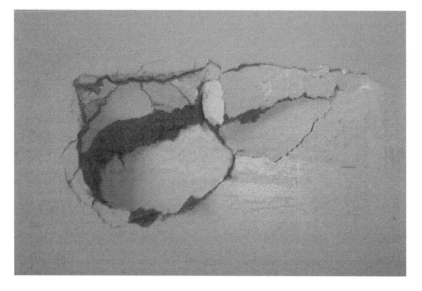

Figure 4.5   Hammer mark made in painted hardboard, which is a typical surface used on many internal doors.

detail that is present (Figure 4.6). If there is any patterning present this should be noted, along with the orientation relative to any edges. The orientation is important as it can give information concerning the direction in which the tool was used to grip the object. If the marks are full width this should be measured and noted, otherwise a minimum width can be given if the marks overlap the edge of the item that has been gripped.

4.2.4   The tool(s)

Having carried out an initial examination of the mark(s) and formed an idea of what the tool(s) responsible should look like, consider opening and examining the questioned tool. In some cases an initial screening can

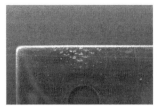 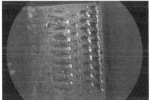 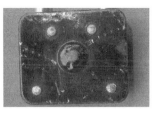

Figure 4.6 A grip mark by a vice (left), locking pliers (middle) and a wrench (right), to demonstrate differences in appearance and class features being considered.

be carried out through the packaging to determine if there are obvious differences, e.g. in size, shape or type of tool, which could preclude the need for further examination, although even this brief examination should be fully recorded in the case notes. This is particularly useful where large numbers of tools have been submitted and it is preferable to limit the number of tools examined in any detail. It is also useful to help identify the most likely tools where DNA or fingerprint examination may be required so that these can be dealt with before doing a detailed comparison. In addition, it can help to think about how much character the tool has and whether you would expect it to leave much detail in the mark.

If the items are opened and contact traces could be a part of the examination, this is best conducted on a different bench than that for the marks' examination and in a different room if possible. Contact traces should be recovered prior to bringing the tool and mark(s) together for any direct comparison. If the marks show reliable features that are different from any of the detail that is present on a tool, the examination can be terminated at this stage. Remember that for various reasons there may be features on the tool that may not be obviously present in the mark; a tool should not necessarily be excluded just because there is a lack of apparent corresponding detail in a mark. A more detailed examination will be needed when a tool cannot be excluded from having made a mark. This is dealt with in Chapter 5. It is useful at this stage to identify and record e.g. different faces of a screwdriver blade or cutting tool, both in case notes and on the tool itself. Any labelling e.g. face A will be used subsequently to identify the relevant areas of the tool used to make test marks that can be compared with marks from the scene.

4.3 Mainly dynamic marks

There are basically two situations where striations are formed, one where a single-bladed tool has slid across a surface and one where a cutting tool has been used to partially or completely cut/sever a piece of material.

4.3.1   Levering marks with striations

The situation where a tool slides across a surface has similarities to the one discussed earlier in this chapter, where the tool has been used as a lever and created an impressed mark. Although the striations in this case may be the most obvious feature to the mark, there could be impressed detail at the point where the tool initially came in contact with the surface before sliding across it. Examine the starting point and look for any evidence to determine whether the tool has rounded, worn corners or sharp, new corners. Also, consider if there is any sign of a bevelled tip bevelling anywhere on the tip or edges of the tool – remember the possibility of an edge of the tool having slipped if the tool twisted while being used (Figure 4.7). Note whether the striae are perpendicular to the starting point; if they are at an angle it shows that the tool blade was at an angle to the direction of movement of the tool. In this case, the length of the starting point will be less than the width of the tool tip and for this reason is sometimes called 'foreshortening' (Figure 4.8). Examine the questioned tool and check that it would be capable of making the mark(s), after which make a decision on whether to examine the striae or the impressed detail first.

4.3.2   Cutting and stabbing marks

There is a wide variety of cutting tools and it would be difficult to classify them all in a meaningful way. The tools that have been most commonly

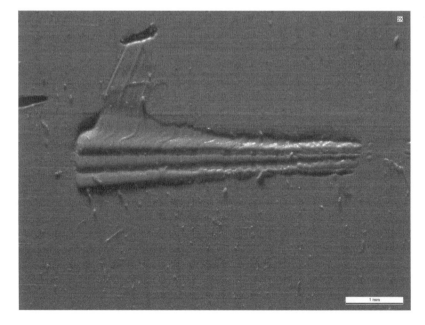

Figure 4.7   Cast of a dynamic mark, shows juddering and twisting of the tool responsible as it slipped across the substrate.

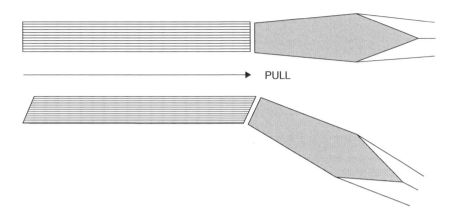

Figure 4.8 Foreshortening effect shown when the tip of a tool is at an angle to direction of travel (bottom), as opposed to being square on (top).

examined by the authors are bolt cutters of various types, side cutters for use in building, fencing and electrical work, heavy-duty electrician's pliers, various types of pipe cutters and knives. The marks made by these tools cover the central features present in the generality of marks left by cutting tools and will be used as examples in the following. For pipe cutters, however, the more significant detail is usually that impressed in marks by damage on either the cutting wheel or rollers.

The first step in the examination is to decide whether the mark has been by a double- or single-bladed tool. With a single-bladed tool each of the cuts will originate from just one side of the cut object (although different cuts may be made from different sides) (Figure 4.9), whereas double-blade cutters will leave marks that originate on both sides at the same time (Figure 4.10).

Single-bladed tools, such as knives, are normally used on relatively soft materials such as brake hose, tyre walls and even blocks of drugs (e.g. cannabis resin) but can also be used on harder materials such as wires. The cuts are usually as a result of trying to sever the object or to cut it into smaller pieces, although those in tyre walls are better thought of as stab marks (stab marks in post-mortem samples are considered in a separate section).

Examine the cut surfaces using low-power microscopy to determine if there is any useful impressed or striated detail present, that deserves further examination. Also, note if contact traces would be expected from the cut object on the tool. For example, the insulation on wires may be of more than one colour and this, if transferred to the tool, together with traces of the copper conductor, may be of more evidential value than the marks present.

When considering tyre stabbings we are usually talking about a variety of actions that can be used to damage a tyre and cause it to deflate. In some cases a knife is pushed into a tyre and then moved sideways to slash the

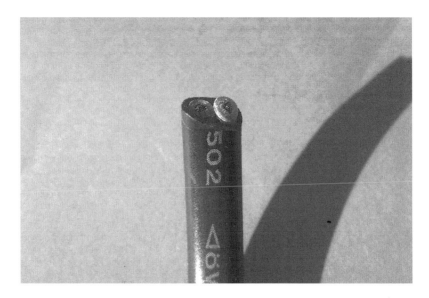

Figure 4.9   Single-bladed cut by cable being held in a loop and a knife pulled through it.

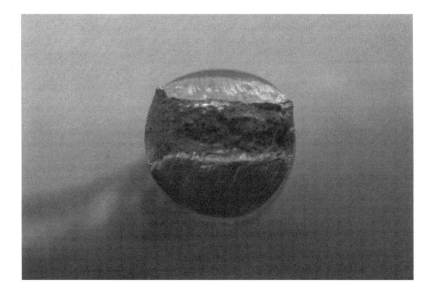

Figure 4.10   Double-bladed cut.

tyre wall causing elongated marks. Most tyre damage, however, is caused by pushing a knife or other pointed object into the tyre then pulling it straight out again. A selection of potential types of implement is shown here. They include not only knives, of various shapes and sizes, but also objects such as nails, bradawls and even screwdrivers.

With either action, most of the characteristic detail will be imparted to the thickness of the rubber as it is cut, but there can also be detail on the outer surface of the tyre that will help with the examination. Indeed, the initial examination of the tyre wall where the implement has been inserted can go a long way to establishing the type of implement that was used. Thus, the initial examination should concentrate on finding *every* area of damage to the tyre by looking at both the outer and inner surfaces. Do not just rely on marks that have been pointed out/marked by the police examiners. They may have finished their examination on finding one or more marks and missed others. Until a detailed laboratory examination is carried out, it is not necessarily possible to say which marks contain the best detail or, potentially, if more than one implement has been used to impart the damage.

At this stage there is no need to cast the marks and such casting may actually obscure detail that has been left on the outer surface. The positions of the areas of damage should be noted on either a drawing or photograph of the tyre. The damage can then be photographed *in situ*. Examination by eye, magnifying lens and bench microscope of the surface around the damage can help to identify the exact shape of the damage, whether it is a single point of entry or elongated. The former would suggest the use of a simple pointed object and the latter would suggest the use of a knife, but at this stage would not necessarily suggest either a stab or a cut. Next, check for bruising, or disturbance of deposits, around the damage. If the object has been inserted deeply into the hole, there may be an impression from the handle end, such as a ferrule. Finally, check the actual shape of the damage, particularly if a knife has been used, which could indicate the shape and condition of the blade. Is the damage straight or ragged? Are the ends sharp and clean or are there 'Y' shapes at either end?

If a tool such as a bradawl has been used, the hole will essentially be small and round. If the ferrule has made contact when the bradawl was fully inserted there may be a ring (annulus) around the hole (Figure 4.11). The diameter of this ring should correspond to that of the ferrule and may contain characteristic detail in the resulting impressed mark.

Nails can also be used and the detail would depend on method of manufacture and shapes of the tips, but typically they have points roughly pyramidal in form. Holes made by these could have four small cuts radiating out from the central point (Figure 4.12).

Most knives, such as kitchen knives, have a blade with one edge sharpened and a flat back (Figure 4.13). The sharpened edge would cut through the rubber leaving a sharply defined end to the cut, but a flat back typically has small cuts (potentially combined with some tearing) at either side in the form of a 'Y' (Figure 4.14). Some types (such as bayonets) have two sharpened edges and both will cut through rubber leaving no 'Y' shapes at the ends (Figure 4.15).

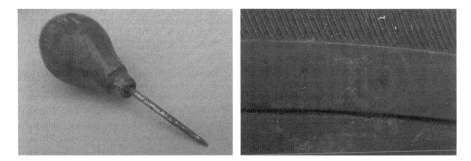

Figure 4.11   A bradawl (left) and a bradawl mark (right), showing the ferrule surrounding a puncture hole.

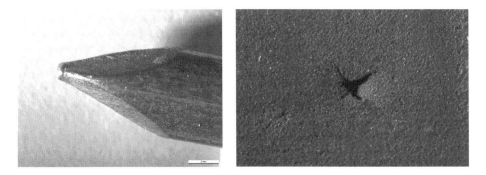

Figure 4.12   Tip of a typical nail (left) and a hole in a tyre made by such a nail (right).

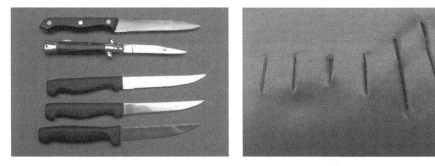

Figure 4.13   Various knives with a flat back (left) and typical stab marks made by such knives in thin metal sheet (right).

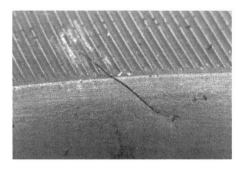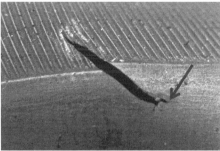

Figure 4.14 Typical 'Y' shape of stab mark made using a flat-backed knife in tyre rubber, relaxed (left) and stretched (right). Top of the 'Y' indicated.

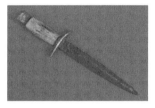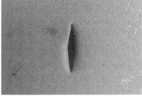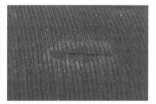

Figure 4.15 A bayonet-type knife (left); stab marks made with it in thin metal (middle) and in tyre rubber (right) show two sharp edges.

The lengths of any damage should be measured as this may relate to the width of the blade responsible, although that depends on the action used and angle of insertion. The outside surface around each area of damage can then be cast to replicate any fine detail.

Bear in mind that damage to a tyre could also be the result of an accidental non-criminal event, for example, running over a nail or broken glass.

It is important at this stage to evaluate carefully the potential evidential value that the marks could provide. Much time and effort can be wasted on a detailed examination of these marks that is not warranted by such detail as is present. Examine the questioned tool in the light of the findings from the mark examination.

Double-bladed cutting tools normally leave a characteristic cut profile in the material (Figures 4.16 and 4.17). The profile can often be determined by the unaided eye and only the lowest power magnification – around ×5 – is needed for this part of the examination. The findings are not definitive, as misaligned blades and poor use of the tool can both give rise to unexpected profiles. If the mark is on a severed padlock shackle and the profile is a fairly straight fracture, check the rest of the shackle and body to determine if there are indications that it has been broken by levering, rather than having been cut. Examine the central part of the cut mark where the blades came to

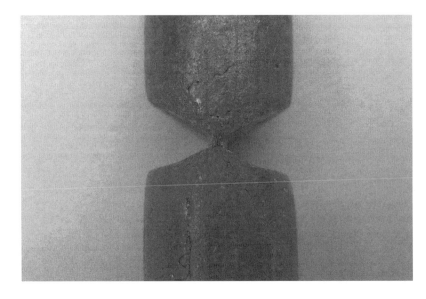

Figure 4.16   A typical profile of a double-bladed cut mark, made in lead rod using bolt cutters.

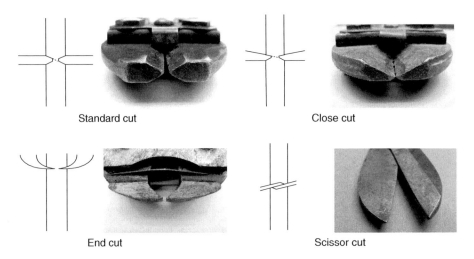

Figure 4.17   Diagram to show different double-bladed cut profiles, depending on the type and set of the cutting blades.

rest and determine if there is characteristic impressed detail present. Decide whether the striation detail in the cut is better than the impressed detail for thorough examination. Note if the impressed detail, together with the striations, suggest that there is gross damage to the tool blades.

Examine the questioned tool and check that it would be capable of generating the profile of the cut. Examine the blades to see if there is smearing

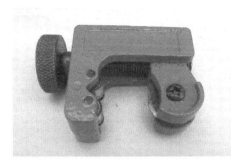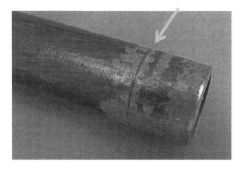

Figure 4.18 A pipe cutter (left) and a pipe with a partial cut mark on it, as indicated, and a fully cut exposed end (right).

or any cleaning of the blades that corresponds to the shape of the cut material. This is not usually important as a contact trace but does indicate the region for later detailed examination after having made a comparison test mark.

Pipe cutters normally work by having a wheel (or series of wheels) that rotates around the circumference of the pipe, gradually cutting through it in a circular motion (Figure 4.18). Check especially for partial cuts, which may reveal the presence of notches and burrs around the cutting edge of the disc. Also look to either side of the cuts (partial or complete) as there may be impressed detail left by the rollers on the pipe cutter (on the opposite side from the cutting disc).

4.4 Saw marks

The examination of a saw mark is based mainly upon detail relating to class and sub-class features rather than individual characteristics. The actions by which marks are left are also different from those for most other types of mark. To help understand saw marks a brief summary of relevant details about saw blades and how they leave marks is given here. This will also be relevant when trying to evaluate the evidence from saw mark examinations.

There are very many different types of saws, including hacksaws, panel saws, tenon saws, pruning saws, circular saws and band saws. Examples of some of the different types of saw available are shown in Figure 4.19. They have different forms of construction, but essentially every saw blade has a series of teeth along the length or around the circumference of the blade. There are two ways in which a saw blade is used to cut a surface. With circular saws and band saws the blade is moved in a single direction. Most hand and power saws use a reciprocating action in which the blade is moved backwards and forward or up and down. Normally, material is only removed from the surface being cut in one direction of action, usually the forward or down stroke if the blade is fitted and used correctly. Each tooth acts like a

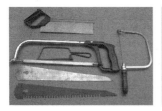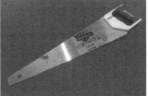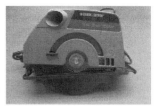

Figure 4.19 Photographs show various different types of saws (left), a panel saw (middle) and circular saw (right).

miniature chisel and leaves its own characteristic detail, but each following tooth then modifies this to varying extents. This makes specific comparison extremely difficult. The individual tooth responsible for making a particular mark would have to be identified and, even then, this would only work if the mark does not contain composite detail from more than one tooth.

Saws for different purposes have different characteristics in respect of tooth size, shape, spacing and set. Traditionally, the spacing of the teeth was expressed in the number of teeth per inch (tpi) (or per 25 mm). For example, hacksaws typically have blades of 18, 24 or 32 tpi, while panel saws may be around 4–8 tpi. The teeth on a single blade are normally of equal size and spacing. Examples of the teeth on panel saws, tenon saws and hacksaws with this regular spacing are shown in Figure 4.20.

There are some saw blades, usually for hacksaws, that have a progressive tooth spacing along the length. Others, such as pruning saws, may have teeth of different size and shape as shown in Figure 4.21. Circular saw blades, as shown in Figure 4.22 generally have evenly spaced teeth, although these are arranged around the circumference of the blade and are usually much wider apart than on most hand saws, or small electric saws.

As well as variations in tooth spacing, looking straight down on the saw blade will show that there are differences in the arrangement of the teeth; the set of the saw blade. Figure 4.23 shows the commonest repeat pattern sets, which are:

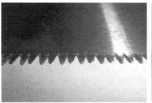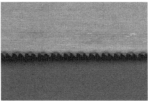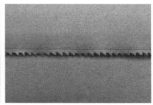

Figure 4.20 A panel saw with a jet cut blade (left), a tenon saw blade with alternate set (middle) and a hacksaw blade with wavy set (right).

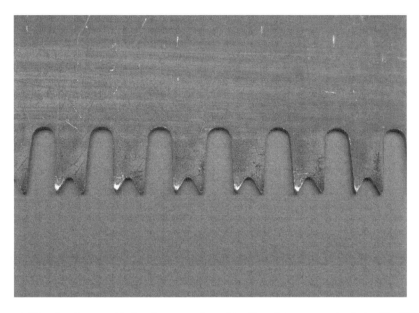

Figure 4.21 Pruning saw blade, shows spacing of teeth points are regular but with differing sizes.

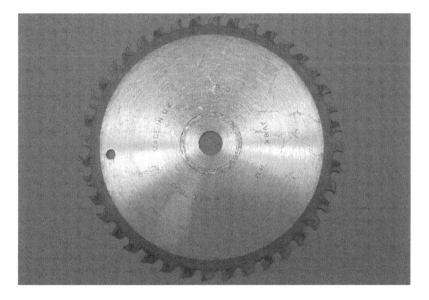

Figure 4.22 Circular saw blade.

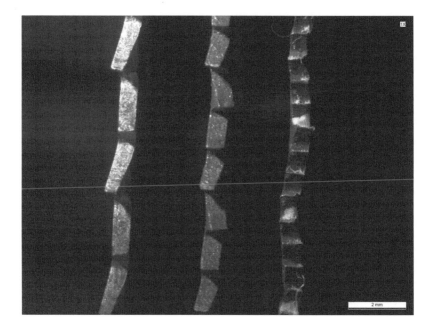

Figure 4.23   Examples of alternate (left), raker (middle) and wavy (right) set blades.

- **alternate** (left): one tooth angled to the right of the blade the next left;

- **raker** (middle): one tooth right, then central, then left, then central;

- **wavy** (right): blade has teeth on a wave-shaped edge.

Another type of set, used on some panel saws is 'jet cut' (as shown in Figure 4.20). This is similar to an alternate set in that every other tooth is very slightly set to one side. The main feature of a jet cut blade is that instead of the teeth being uniform in thickness (corresponding to the main body of the blade) each tooth has sharpened, bevelled edges (similar to a chisel). The side that is sharpened alternates along the blade.

A general examination of the questioned item with the unaided eye will normally reveal whether it has been cut with a saw. The mark may have some or all of the characteristics shown in Figure 4.24. Use a microscope, starting at a low magnification of about ×10 to determine if there is any useful characteristic detail present. External oblique lighting is essential for this, as there is only shallow relief in any wave pattern left by the saw teeth. If the features cannot be clearly seen on the original item, casting the mark usually helps, especially if the detail is recessed, but casting should not be done until the cut areas have been examined for contact trace materials (especially paint).

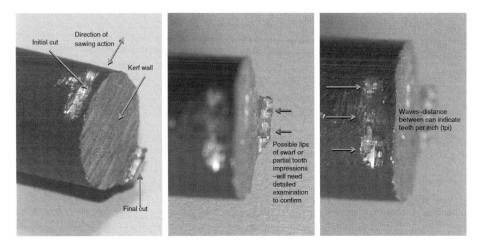

Figure 4.24 Saw mark features – shape of initial cut and regular parallel fine striations indicate a straight blade with sharp teeth and no change of direction of operation of the saw. In this case, the saw is an 18 tpi hacksaw blade.

It is often difficult to begin a saw cut and this can result in the blade jumping from one position to another, leaving a partial cut in the material. Likewise, at the end of the cut the material can break leaving a lip. These initial and final cuts can provide a great deal of information and should be examined carefully.

If the edges of an initial cut have a dumbbell shape (as shown in Figure 4.25), rather than being parallel, this indicates a distorted/damaged blade, although it can also be the result of poor sawing technique. If due to poor technique, the lines at the bottom of the mark will normally be at an angle to the main direction of the cut.

Measure the width of the cut (the kerf), which will depend on various factors. These include the thickness of the metal forming the blade and how the saw teeth have been set. It is not just the type of set that affects the kerf width, but also how far the teeth have been moved over from the centre line of the blade.

Although a wavy set blade (as previously shown in Figure 4.23) superficially involves the greatest lateral displacement of the teeth it does not necessarily give a wider kerf than an alternate or raker set blade, which may have larger (and longer) teeth, such that the outer tips of teeth are further apart. The wavy set is usually found on the blades with the finest teeth (usually 32 tpi). These are often, but not exclusively, intended for use with the smaller hacksaw frames (junior or midget hacksaws). The set may be best determined by examining the appearance of the bottom of the cut. If there are two or three clearly separate lines of marks, parallel to the edges of the cut, this supports the inference that the blade has an alternate or raker set, whereas a

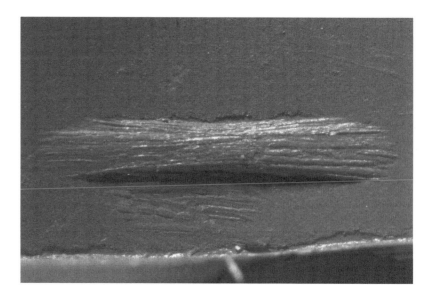

Figure 4.25   Cast of a dumbbell shaped mark made with a damaged/twisted blade.

large number of fine lines supports a wavy set. A jet cut blade will often leave partial cuts that have a raised V shape in the centre caused by the chamfering on the edges of the teeth.

There may also be partial impressions or other details to indicate the tooth spacing. Figure 4.26 shows a cast of various partial cuts in a rod. The upper mark shows two lines across the mark (at the right-hand end) indicating the positions of two adjacent teeth, one towards one side of the cut and one towards the other. This suggests the use of an alternate set blade, while the spacing between them (of approximately 2.4 mm) would suggest that the blade has approximately 10–11 tpi. The second mark is narrower, with many fine lines along it. This suggests a hacksaw blade with a wavy set. The teeth marks just to the left of centre are approximately 1 mm apart and suggest the blade has 24 tpi.

Most commercial hacksaw blades intended for use with a standard size frame are coloured, often with one base colour and details printed in another. Different manufacturers will normally use various combinations of colour. Plate 8 shows a variety of hacksaw blades illustrating this.

Thus, the examiner should check if there is coloured paint smeared on the cut surface. An initial examination of the colour(s) can be useful to either eliminate a blade that has been submitted for examination or to indicate the brand and type of blade used. While contamination from the surface on which the paint was recovered may cause some problems with the interpretation of analytical results from these types of paint smear, detailed physical and chemical comparison can be useful, as different batches of

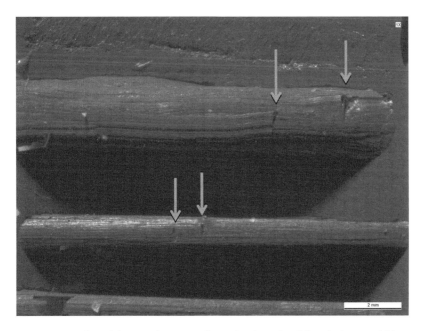

Figure 4.26 Cast of partial cuts. The two main marks show detail in relation to width, set and tooth spacing (indicated by arrows), as described in the text.

paint used by a single manufacturer may be of slightly different shades and chemical composition.

Check the submitted saw blade to determine whether on the information gathered so far the blade could have been used to cut the item. This should be done through the packaging if possible as any that are not eliminated at this stage should be checked for contact trace material before carrying out any detailed comparison with the scene marks. At the very least, this initial examination should be carried out in DNA clean conditions if there is a possibility that there may be traces of body material on the saw used or if ownership is disputed and may have to be confirmed by checking for the handler's DNA on the tool.

4.5 Post-mortem samples

In dealing with post-mortem samples, there may be various types of marks to be considered. In dismemberment cases these are likely to be some form of cut marks on the bones, usually caused by either a saw or a chopping action (although there may also be score marks around the bone if the flesh has been cut through to expose the bone). If a blunt object has been used to hit someone, there may be impressed marks on the bones. In cases of stabbing, there may be impressions from the tip of a tool if it has hit the surface of the bone or there could be slicing marks if the knife has passed between the ribs, for example cutting into them.

As well as examining the marks themselves, the case circumstances and other information obtained at the time of submission, the pathologist's report and post-mortem photographs should also be used to obtain the best picture as to what has happened and what type of marks may be found. The pathologist will normally have made an assessment of soft tissue wounds and will have considered what type of implement may have caused damage to cartilage and bone. The scientist could use these assessments, but will mainly be concerned with looking at finer detail in the marks through cartilage or bone. In most cases, the basic initial examination probably falls within one of the categories described earlier in this chapter, but an additional problem is to prepare the sample for examination. For a tool mark examiner who is not an anatomist there are lots of anatomy/bone textbooks that could be used to visualise how and where the submitted bone would lie in the body, as could access to a human skeleton (or a good model of one). One example of a useful textbook is *Gray's Anatomy*, which was first published in 1858 (Standring, 2008).

It is important to remember that all pathology samples represent a health hazard and need proper facilities for examination. A minimum requirement is a designated biological grade fume cupboard that can be washed and sterilised after use. Wearing personal protective equipment (PPE) is mandatory. A laboratory coat and gloves should be worn at all times to handle the item and a biological hazard disposal bin must be located close to the examination area. Depending on the sample, a facemask or protective eye glasses may also be needed.

It may not be possible to carry out a microscopic examination within the fume cupboard so a bench area should also be prepared close by. Such samples tend to be quite messy. Whilst health and safety is paramount for the examiner and those working around them, one also needs to also remember that the samples can be a potential source of DNA contamination, so location of the examination needs to be considered carefully. Again, as mentioned in Chapter 3, it is important to remember that you are dealing with human body tissue and it should be treated with respect and in compliance with local legislation covering such materials.

Before proceeding too far into preparing and cleaning the samples, the surfaces of both the flesh and bone around the tool marks should be examined for contact traces. This is especially important where the use of a saw or an axe is suspected, as the blades are often painted and traces of that can form a significant part of the examination. Indeed, it is possible that flakes of paint recovered from the item can be physically fitted back to the tool from which it originated.

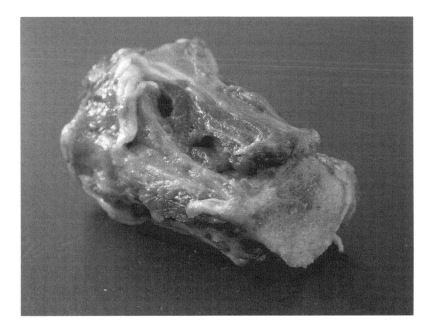

Figure 4.27 Bone sample with a sawn end, as it might look when received.

Figure 4.27 shows a bone sample as it might look when submitted[1]; the pathologist must be careful not to cut down to the bone or cause any unnecessary damage. The first stage is to remove as much flesh as possible before using an enzyme to clean the bone surface. For this a non-metal tool should be used, such as plastic forceps or a wooden scraper. A wooden scraper can be made from a drinks stirrer or lolly stick; a wooden knife like implement can be bought from art suppliers that deal in clay and ceramic materials. In some cases this will expose the mark sufficiently that it can be cast. Casting at this stage must be considered if the mark is partly in cartilage as the following cleaning process can partially or completely digest the cartilage destroying the mark and detail within it. Likewise, restrictions may be imposed in terms of both time and what processes can be carried out[2] and this could mean that casting without cleaning off the flesh is the only option. It will be necessary to degrease the mark with alcohol before trying to take the cast and to sterilise the cast after it has been removed from the mark.

If it is not possible to cast the mark from the partially defleshed item, the remaining flesh is removed by digesting with an enzyme solution. The

---

[1] Please note that where we talk about marks in bone and cartilage throughout this book, none of the associated images are from a human body for reasons of sensitivity. The images are of marks in animal bone (or a human skeleton model as in Chapter 3).

[2] For instance, by the need to have the item restored in time for a funeral or if the items need to be restored in a condition as close as possible to that in which they were submitted.

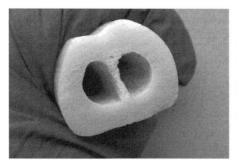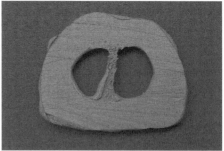

Figure 4.28   A cleaned up bone (left), and a cast taken from the sawn end (right).

easiest to obtain are those used in biological washing powders, alcalase being one example. The enzyme is made up in a buffered solution, in the case of alcalase a phosphate buffer at pH 5, the item then immersed in it and the whole system placed in a thermostatic bath held at a temperature of around 30–40 °C. This is the safest method and gives the most control over what happens to the item. This can be left overnight to deflesh but may require up to a few days. Biological washing powders themselves can also be used, but while these are convenient they are intended for removing stains not digesting large amounts of flesh. Near room temperature, biological washing powders act very slowly on this type of sample and the temptation is to raise the temperature to nearer the boiling-point of water. This results in the loss of collagen from the bone, potentially altering the bone structure as well as making it more brittle. The same criticism applies to autoclaving the item as received in water. While after autoclaving the flesh is easily removed from the bone, there is the possibility of altering the structure of the bones.

After removing the flesh and leaving a clean bone, any marks present can again be examined under the microscope. The cleaned up marks can also be cast at this stage and examined for relevant detail. Figure 4.28 shows the end of a bone after it has been cleaned and sterilised and then cast. As with all types of tool mark, a cast is usually taken to see the detail more easily, and to allow it to be viewed under a comparator.

4.6   Alphanumeric punches

There are basically two types of punch encountered in tool mark examinations.

- Those used to sink a character into a metal or other fixed substrate (typically vehicle engine blocks or high-value equipment where the original identification has either been altered or replaced). This utilises sets of individual metal punches with mirror images of alphanumeric characters on one end that are struck into the surface leaving an impression of that character (Figure 4.29).

- Those used on portable plastic substrates (typically credit cards and similar items as well as marking tapes e.g. Dymo™). This utilises embossing machines of various types. In these machines all the alphanumeric characters are present with different ones being presented to the surface to be embossed as required. There are usually two punches for each character: a raised punch (of the letter/number required) pushes up from the rear of the substrate and leaves a recessed negative impression of the character, while a recessed 'punch' of the same character is held against the front of the substrate and leaves a raised positive impression of the character (Figure 4.30).

For both types the characters come in a range of styles and sizes (as shown in Figure 4.31), with some variation in the specific shapes between sets of the same basic style.

The punch marks from fixed objects are normally submitted as casts from the original items and may not be of the highest quality, especially if the original surface was dirty. While it is always sensible to check any repeat characters to help identify common features, it is a necessary part of an examination of this type if it is suspected that the cast is less than perfect. Ideally, duplicate casts will have been taken for each set of marks and later casts may show the detail more clearly as the first has cleaned the surface. Check the size and style of the characters against the known set(s) of punches submitted. Bear in mind that not all of the relevant punches may be available

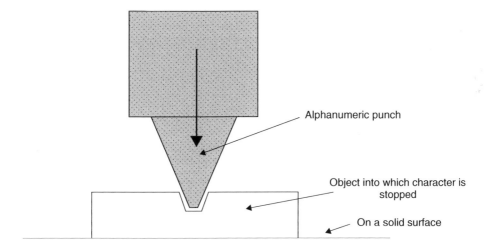

Figure 4.29 Showing how an alphanumeric punches stamp numbers into a surface.

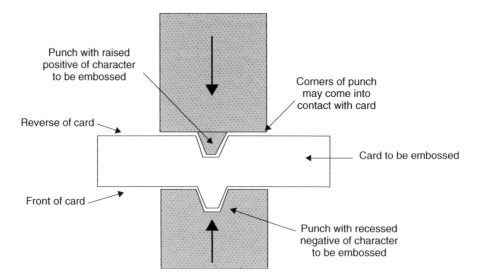

Figure 4.30   Demonstrating embossing characters on a credit card.

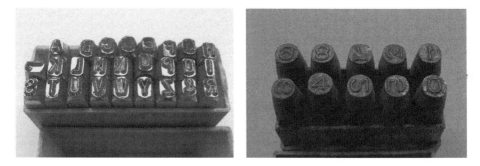

Figure 4.31   Typical sets of letter punches, including '&' (left) and number punches (right). As the '6' and '9' are interchangeable, some sets may only include one of these.

or that punches from more than one set may have been used to produce the new number.

The marks examined in portable substrates such as credit cards will need to have both sides examined for suitable detail, although at the initial stage this may not be necessary. With marking tapes, the machine involved is normally small enough to be transported to the laboratory. With plastic cards, most modern machinery is transportable and should be relatively easy to examine in the laboratory, but in some instances the comparisons may involve using known marks made outside the laboratory. Whereas it is relatively easy to compare casts of punched numbers from fixed objects against the original punches, this is not possible for machine-produced numbers. The characters are integral in the machine and the appearance of the 'crime' characters can be influenced by the thickness of the card or tape on which they were produced. The examination of the cards is best achieved by making test cards in the machine, so a supply of similar cards is advisable. It is also necessary to check at an early stage that the machinery (especially as it is likely to be electrically powered) is safe to use. Once the test cards have been produced using the relevant characters, the embossed characters on both the front and reverse of crime and test cards should be cast. Again check the size and style of the questioned and known marks and also see if there is any potentially characteristic detail present.

4.7   Using tool marks for intelligence purposes

As part of the initial examination of tool marks recovered from scenes of crime, an assessment will have been made about the type of tool used and potential detail within those marks. This information can be used in various ways to provide intelligence information for the investigators, through:

1. information about the type and size of tool(s) used;

2. scene-to-scene linking without a tool;

3. scene-to-scene linking using a tool recovered from a scene;

4. linking suspect's tool(s) to previously unsuspected scenes.

4.7.1   Type and size of tool

While it may not be possible to obtain much information about the tool(s) used at a scene, even minimal information can be invaluable to investigators. It must be as accurate as possible, giving suggestions as to the type of tool responsible whenever possible. 'A screwdriver with a blade 9 mm wide at the tip, with the blade tapering towards the tip and grinding detail running across the blade', not just 'a screwdriver', is preferable, but obviously depends on what information can be clearly obtained from the marks.

While this type of information for the screwdriver would cover a large number of tools that could be recovered from suspects, the use of a more specialist tool may point the investigators in a particular direction.

4.7.2   Scene-to-scene linking without a tool

Tool marks lend themselves to scene-to-scene comparison, with the potential of obtaining specific links. Marks from different locations can be screened against each other to see if any have been made by the same tool. In order for the marks to be comparable, they also have to have been made by the same part of the tool used. The first point to check is whether or not a tip width is present. If the marks are clearly made by tools of different widths there is no point in continuing, but if they have been made by the same width (and type) of tool it is worth looking at any fine detail that is present.

For impressed marks there may be characteristic detail present that can be compared in the same way as scene marks against test marks from a tool. Full width marks are not necessary – for example there may be just an impression from the corner of a tool present where beading has been levered from a window. It is not the quantity, but quality of the mark that is important.

For sliding marks, if the same face of the tool has been used at a similar angle then a detailed comparison can again be carried out. Check the full lengths of all sliding marks as they may have been made by different parts of the tool or at different angles.

When reporting scene-to-scene comparisons it is important to remember that the same tool can leave marks that cannot be matched with each other because either different parts of the tool have been used or the tool may have been modified between the two offences. Not finding a link is not the same as saying different tools have been used, it is just that there is no intelligence/evidence to say that the marks were made by the same tool.

4.7.3   Scene-to-scene linking using a tool recovered from a scene

In some cases a tool may have been recovered from the scene of a crime. Even if the tool cannot be associated with a suspect, it can be compared with marks from earlier scenes to establish whether or not it was used at those scenes; there may be other evidence at one of these that can be linked to a suspect.

4.7.4   Linking suspect's tool(s) to previously unsuspected scenes

It goes without saying that if suspects are arrested for an offence and have tools that can be associated with them, those tools can be compared with earlier offences to establish if they have been used at any of them.

4.7.5   Setting up a database

In addition to carrying out these examinations following specific requests, centralised databases can be produced where information about the offences and the marks recovered from them can be stored, indexed and searched. One such database was run by the Metropolitan Police Forensic Science Laboratory from 1977, originally using edge punch Anson cards that were searched manually, as described by Davis in a 1981 paper. Later, a computerised database was set up. Whatever system is used, the basic information to be stored includes the address and date of the offence and as much information as possible about the tools used that can be gathered from the marks. For the latter this should include an assessment of the size and type of each tool represented in the marks along with an assessment of the quality of the detail present, including information about any potentially useful characteristic detail, such as grinding detail or damage. The best point at which to record the width of the tool is at the tip, as this should be constant, whereas widths vary along the length of a tapering or widening blade. Even if there are only partial marks present it may be possible to obtain a minimum width and to determine if the blade has acute, obtuse or right angled corners, which would suggest it tapers or widens towards the tip or is parallel sided.

The database could also be expanded to include much more information about the scene, such as the type of premises, point(s) of attack, property targeted (type and value) and other specific features of the *modus operandi* (MO) that could be used as additional screening parameters if a search on tool type (e.g. a 9 mm screwdriver) produced a large number of potential marks to look through.

References

Davis, R.J. (1981) An intelligence approach to footwear marks and toolmarks. *Journal of the Forensic Science Society*, **21** (3), 183–193.

Standring, S. (ed.) (2008). *Gray's Anatomy: The Anatomical Basis of Clinical Practice*, 40th edn, Churchill Livingstone, Edinburgh.

5
Detailed Laboratory Examination

5.1 First considerations

While it is a self-evident statement, it is none the less important to realise that the course of the detailed examination will depend on what equipment is available. The importance lies in the fact that very few tool mark laboratories will have all of the possible equipment available; it is just not cost effective. This often generates two different outcomes. When successfully using the equipment for the types of examination that it is best suited to, examiners gain experience that produces better results. This, in turn, feeds back as good results for the submitting authority and often results in more of that type of examination. The other aspect comes about when marks unsuited to the equipment are examined and poor results are obtained. This leads to fewer cases of that type being submitted, with the consequent loss of experience and development.

To some extent this situation can be overcome due to developments in instrument manufacture. Modern scientific instruments have to be designed so that they can be used by a number of different groups of specialists, in order to provide a sufficiently large sales base for commercial success. One method of achieving this is to make the specific instrument from modular components. This places a heavy responsibility on the person tasked with buying the instrumentation, as they will have to specify the individual modules. For example, if photography is to be a routine procedure when using a conventional comparator (which it really should, as it is the best means of recording details of the comparison), then lighting, type of stage holding the items and numerical apertures of the objective lenses all need to be considered and kept

The Forensic Examination and Interpretation of Tool Marks, First Edition.
David Baldwin, John Birkett, Owen Facey and Gilleon Rabey.
© 2013 John Wiley & Sons, Ltd. Published 2013 by John Wiley & Sons, Ltd.

compatible with the photographic system. It is, however, possible to develop a single system that can carry out most of the examinations given below.[1]

5.2   Presentation of material to the comparator

A pre-requisite to carrying out a detailed comparison is to ensure that the comparator is properly balanced by performing an appropriate balance check, as described in Chapter 1.

The tool mark and the test mark will nearly always be in different materials and so the surfaces of the marks potentially have different reflectivities. Although that is not in itself necessarily a problem, in some cases this can cause severe difficulties. With the advent of opaque silicone casting materials with medium reflectivity, it was soon realised that they could be used to cast test marks as well as scene marks. Thus, a direct comparison between the two casts was not only possible but preferable to comparing scene and test marks directly although, even then, for some materials the casts may need to be coated (e.g. by vacuum deposition of a thin metal coating) to see detail at its best.

The following paragraphs give details of how representations of the scene mark and tool/test mark can be combined for use on the comparator. The terms used can be defined as:

- **original scene mark**: an item bearing marks recovered directly from the scene;

- **original cast**: a cast taken of the marks at the scene;

- **original tool**: self-explanatory, being the actual tool seized for comparison;

- **cast**: taken directly from a scene mark, test mark or tool, which will show a mirror image of the detail;

- **replica cast**: a cast (usually) made in the laboratory by taking a cast of the original scene mark, cast or tool with an intermediary compound (such as Permlastic™) and then recasting that with a silicone rubber compound that is suitable for use on a comparator, which will show the detail in the same orientation, and may also be known as a 'recast'.

When presenting marks on a comparator you need to be comparing like with like. A cast taken from a scene mark or from a test mark produces a reversed impression of the mark. For marks comprising striations, the casts of the scene mark and test mark can be compared against each other as they

---

[1] Details of the requirements for a comparator have been given in Chapter 1.

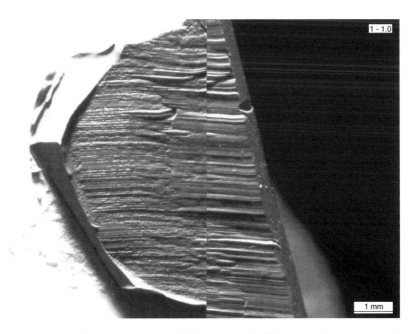

Figure 5.1 A cast of a cut scene mark (left), compared with a cast of a test cut mark made using the suspect tool (right). Note that the cutting edge of the tool in both halves of the image is pointing to the right.

are in the same orientation (Figure 5.1). With impressed marks, details in these casts will correspond directly to the original tool and again these casts can also be compared one with the other.

If the submitted casts of the scene marks have been made in a suitable material they can be used on the comparator and be compared directly with the casts of test marks made in the laboratory. Problems arise when the submitted casts of scene marks are not suitable for use on the comparator. In this instance, a replica cast can be made of the original cast as given above.

Casts of impressed marks can be compared with either casts of test marks or with recasts of a tool, or even directly with the tool. It is often quicker to compare an impressed mark with a test mark, for example by using a screwdriver tip to make an impressed test mark in modelling/dental wax and then casting it, rather than making a replica cast of the tool. In some cases, however, a recast of the relevant part of the tool may show detail more clearly and make the comparison easier (Figure 5.2). Although the impressed mark could be compared directly with the tool, this is unlikely to be done because of difficulties in manipulating the tool on the comparator and differences in reflectivity.

In some cases detail is easier to light and visualise on the original item (or a replica cast of it) and this can be compared with a cast taken directly from the tool using a suitable silicone rubber compound.

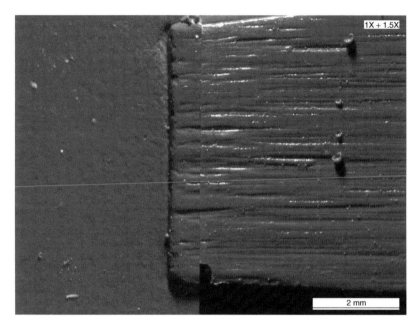

Figure 5.2   A cast of an impressed scene mark, made by a levering tool, compared with a replica cast of the suspect screwdriver, with the tip of both pointing to the left.

When making replica casts from a tool (or from many submitted casts that are not opaque), Permlastic™ can normally be used as the intermediary casting material, as given above. It is, however, incompatible with Isomark™ casting material, on which it does not cure properly, but it can be used to recast from other silicone rubbers. It can also be used when making replicas where the examination involves the physical fit of one part to another. Although it is not often necessary to recast from casts made in Isomark, when needed, modelling/dental wax, described in the next section for use in making test marks, has been used. The wax is melted using a hotplate and painted onto the Isomark cast with a small artist's brush to slowly build up a sheet of wax, from which the Isomark cast can be peeled. This method reduces the formation of bubbles in the wax cast.

Details of the requirements for casting materials are given in Chapter 1 and these materials are generally suitable for taking casts in the laboratory as well as at scenes. However, in the laboratory certain materials and techniques that are unsuitable for use at scenes may be used more effectively. For example, if the mark is likely to trap air, then the item bearing the mark together with the casting material can be placed in a vacuum desiccator to help the removal of the air. Another method of ensuring good contact between the casting material and the surface to be cast is to apply the casting material with a small paintbrush or sharp end of a toothpick while viewing under a microscope. These techniques can be used for credit card numbers, fractured surfaces and similar marks. The slower curing, more fluid, grades of casting materials, such as Isomark™, are useful for casting marks that are inside lock keyways for example.

5.3 Impressed marks

Where the initial examination shows that there is some correspondence, or at least shows no obvious, significant discrepancies[2] between the scene of crime mark and the tool submitted, a detailed comparison is required to confirm or eliminate the tool from having made the mark. The first requirement for the detailed examination is to prepare both items so that the examination is possible. In theory the scene mark does not present much of a problem, in that a cast of some sort will be used, even though in practice it may be difficult to prepare such a cast. Dealing with the tool is more of a problem.

While the impressed scene of crime mark is a direct imprint of the tool, the problem is to estimate how accurately the mark represents the tool. In some cases the representation can be very accurate, in which case a cast of the relevant part of the tool can be directly compared with the cast from the scene tool mark. As mentioned earlier, this would normally mean making a replica cast of the tool for side by side comparison, rather than by trying to manipulate the tool on the comparator. More commonly, the material in which the scene mark is made will not take an accurate impression of all the detail present on the tool.

While the scene mark may not include all of the detail that is present on the tool, comparisons are again often carried out by using replica casts of the blade without the need for test marks. If necessary, test marks could be made in a material similar to that containing the crime mark and a cast taken of these. There are two reasons for this approach: firstly, that it makes the comparison considerably more direct and simpler to evaluate; and secondly, that by examining the test marks it is possible to determine which features are reliably reproduced when the tool is forced into the material. It will also take some account of any relaxation process that takes place after the tool is removed and the material recovers from the pressure applied, which will make it closer to the form of the scene mark.

A range of materials should be kept that can be used in making test marks. What is needed are materials that have the same type of properties as those commonly submitted to the laboratory bearing tool marks and, which, in addition, are unlikely to cause damage to the tool in the process of making test marks. Materials such as painted blocks of wood, offcuts of uPVC window or door frames, modelling/dental wax and lead sheet will provide a range that covers most needs.

---

[2] The correspondence may be very limited. For example, the mark may show just an edge of the tool responsible and the tool has at least one similar edge.

To make test levering marks it is useful to have a workshop vice available. Two pieces of test material are loosely clamped between the jaws, the tool inserted between them and pressure applied to form a levering mark. In this way an impression is obtained both of the tip and the back mark; check with the scene notes to ensure that the test back mark has the same spatial relation to the tip impression as that from the scene. Even if the scene mark comprises just a tip impression or a back impression, two pieces of test material should still be used. Firstly, the second piece prevents the other face of the tool from coming into contact with hard jaws of the vice, potentially damaging it. Secondly, it also allows marks to be made with both faces of the tool (tip and back) by pushing the tool in both directions.

For gripping tools, test marks can be made in sheets of lead or modelling/dental wax. These are usually sufficient if a thin object has been gripped, such as a sheet of metal held in a vice, but many objects that have been gripped are much wider, for example EuroProfile™ door locks (an example of which is shown in Figure 3.9 in Chapter 3). The actual area of the jaws that comes into contact with the surface can be affected by this as they are not usually parallel and differences in pressure will mean that the marks are impressed to a different extent. In these circumstances, the lead sheet can be wrapped round a solid object (such as a block of wood or metal rod) of suitable size so that the jaws are gripping a surface of similar size and shape to the scene item. To locate the area of the vice jaws that potentially made the marks, look at the geometries of the vice and the item that has been gripped. This should establish that the item could not be held in certain orientations. Consideration should also be given here as to the reason why the item had been held in the vice. If it had been held to enable it to be sawn, the item is likely to have projected out horizontally from the jaws, while an object being filed is likely to project from the upper surfaces of the jaws. Having located the most obvious location on the jaws, test marks or casts can be made with those areas.

Impact marks are more difficult with regard to making suitable test marks. The angle at which the impacting tool was used can be highly variable and difficult to reproduce. It is best to start with a mark made by using the tool square on to a sheet of lead or modelling/dental wax, so that an impression of, for example, the whole hammer head is obtained. If an area of particular interest is then identified further test marks can be made by hitting the sheet at a suitable angle with the tool.

Refer to the labelling applied in the initial examination and either take a cast/replica cast from the tool or make test marks with it; label these for future reference, including which aspect of the tool was used. If a test mark was made, take a cast from it and label it. The scene cast (or replica cast taken from it if necessary) and test cast can then be mounted on the stages of the comparator using a material such as plasticine or Blu-Tack™. Starting with the lowest magnification and as broad an illumination as possible, bring both marks into focus using a combination of the height adjustment for the comparator bridge and the item stages. This is the opposite of the normal practice in microscopy. This is because, unlike conventional optical microscopy, it is not possible to prepare the item so that the area to be examined is essentially flat. When moving to a higher magnification adjusting the focus is normally required and this is best done by using the z-axis adjustment of the stage. Using a combination of modifying the item's tilt with the stage mounting material and tilt of the stage head, get the surface to be examined as perpendicular as possible to the optic axis of the comparator bridge objective. The surface to be examined should stay in focus when the $x-y$ translation adjustments are used.

Rotate the stage and use the $x-y$ translation to bring the area of interest into view in the split field shown by the comparator objectives. If a focusing method is present on the lighting system, narrow the illuminating beam down to the area of interest on both the scene cast and the comparison cast. The illumination should normally be at a low angle of incidence to bring the surface detail on the casts into relief, with the angle of incidence and direction being approximately the same for both scene and test casts. The lighting angle (in both the horizontal and vertical planes) should be adjusted to show the detail to its best, but in many cases not all of the detail is clearly visible with just one setting for the lighting. It may be necessary to continue manipulating the marks and the lighting to obtain the best out of different areas of the marks. It is now possible to check if the characteristic features present match in position and morphology in both casts.

Figure 5.3 shows a cast of an impressed scene mark on the left and a replica cast from a suspect tool, as seen in a typical split field view from a comparator. The scale bar indicates the low magnification being used, the vertical dimension representing about 8 mm of the respective casts in real life. A low magnification is being used so that the maximum number of characteristic features can be seen at the same time. Each feature should not only agree in shape but also in position relative to each other and to the edges of the tool, where this can be seen. Depending on the model of comparator being used, there may be devices that can further aid the comparison. In most models it is possible to move the line dividing the two fields so that the continuity of the features can more readily be examined. In some cases it is possible to overlay the two fields, so that each image fills the field of view but one is on top of the other. Some other examples of the different types of detail seen in impressed marks are shown in Figure 5.4.

Most comparators can be fitted with camera systems to record the images. Whenever possible, images of the comparison should be taken as a record of the examination. These can be simply direct photographs showing the image of the scene and test marks side by side as viewed through the comparator. Equipment that is more modern is fitted with digital cameras that are linked to a computer. This allows images to be stored electronically (using an auditable

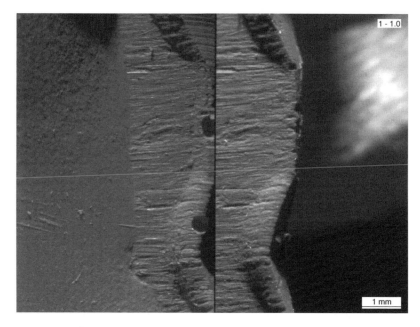

Figure 5.3   Cast of an impressed scene mark made by a cutting tool (left), compared with a replica cast of the suspect bolt cutter blade (right).

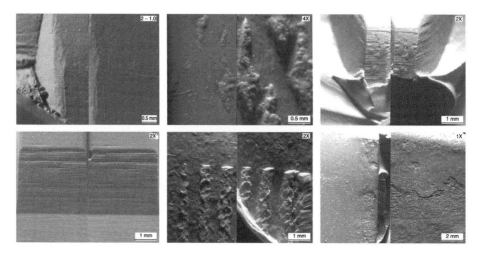

Figure 5.4   Series of photographs to show casts of impressed scene marks (left half of each image) and either a replica cast of the suspect tool or a cast from a test mark made by it (right half of each image).

program). If a series of photographs have been taken of different areas of the mark, using different lighting conditions, a selection of these can be printed out for inclusion in the case notes (and even in reports). Some of the computer programs have the facility to stitch together a series of images taken along the length of marks that are too big to include in a single image, so that all of the detail can be seen together. An indication should be given as to the orientation of the tool and mark.

It is possible to dispense with the comparator altogether and use a macro photographic set-up for this type of examination. In this case, both the scene mark and the test item are photographed at the same scale; a scale should be included in the image. One is printed on photographic paper and the other on transparent film and the two can be directly compared by overlays. There can be problems where the mark is not on a nearly flat surface or where very small detail is involved.

When determining the level of correspondence between the scene mark and the test mark, it is just as important to note dissimilarities as similarities. Even though the tool submitted for examination has the correct class features and a similar degree of wear to the tool making the scene mark, if the microscopic features show significant discrepancies, then it was not the tool that made the mark. If there are some apparent differences and some similarities then some explanation of the apparent differences is needed before accepting that the tool may have been responsible for the mark. This may come from the details provided in the documentation.

For example, a number of marks were made at the scene and the mark examined was one of the earlier ones made, with the tool being modified as it made subsequent marks. In this case, detailed examination of other marks from the scene (if submitted) may show this modification. If there was a time interval between the marks being made and the tool being discovered, the tool may have been used or otherwise damaged (e.g. by being dropped) in that period. The information, together with the mark itself, may also suggest that the scene mark was made in a specific way and this needs to copied more accurately to reproduce the same detail in the tests. It is also possible that the material used for making the test impression was not sufficiently close to the scene mark material. It is important to keep notes of the attempts to understand and settle any apparently significant differences, particularly if they have not have been resolved after making further test marks.

5.4 Marks with striations

A detailed examination of a mark showing striations will, of necessity, involve making test marks and this is the most difficult part of the examination. The reason for this is not difficult to understand. Most of the striae used for the comparison have a width in the range of tens to hundreds of microns so that the appearance of the tool at the scale of microns needs to be considered. At this scale, edges and surfaces appear rounded rather than rectangular and flat. Further, the surfaces are uneven and have micron-sized projections present, which give rise to the striations seen in the tool mark. However, a small change in the angle and pressure that the working edge of the tool has with the surface will alter which of the projections are in contact with the surface. Hence, the appearance of the tool mark is very sensitive to how it has been made. Ultimately, it is not the size of the features that is important, but how characteristic they are and how well they can be visualised and compared.

As we have already discussed in Chapter 1, in general terms there are four main types of action that produce striated marks. These are: sliding marks, for example, where a tool slips across the surface; cutting marks, either where a single-bladed tool such as a knife slices through an object or where a double-bladed tool is used to sever an object; and stabbing marks, where a tool is forced into a material. These need to be dealt with in slightly different ways and therefore will be considered separately below. Other striated marks can be produced by actions such as drilling and sawing. These generally fit into the described categories, but are also dealt with separately later in this chapter.

5.4.1   Sliding marks

This type of mark is often encountered on surfaces such as metal, plastic and painted wood (sometimes even on unpainted wood), as well as other less commonly encountered materials. Suitable materials for test marks are lead sheet and sheets of modelling/dental wax. Before making the test marks, read all the background information regarding where the mark was found and how it might have been made, then correlate this with the information obtained from the preliminary examination, so that consideration can be given to making the test mark in as close a way as possible to the scene mark. It is also important to note whether the mark was made as the tool was being used to lever open the object (a levering mark) or as the tool was inserted into the object (a push mark). As well as the direction in which the tool was used, the information in the documentation and the initial examination of the mark may indicate the angle to the vertical at which the tool was used. In many cases it may not be possible to determine exactly how the tool was used and it may be necessary to make test marks using both actions. However, it is often preferable to start by making levering type marks and compare these, only going on to make push marks if no specific link has been found.

For a general levering mark, where there is not much information, it is often useful to start out by making a test mark with the tool starting out at a low angle but increasing the angle so that the tool ends in an almost vertical position (see Figure 5.5). This will cover most of the options for the angle of the tool to the material being levered.

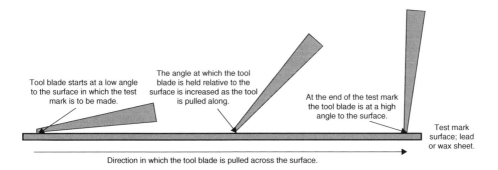

Tool blade starts at a low angle to the surface in which the test mark is to be made.

The angle at which the tool blade is held relative to the surface is increased as the tool is pulled along.

At the end of the test mark the tool blade is at a high angle to the surface.

Test mark surface; lead or wax sheet.

Direction in which the tool blade is pulled across the surface.

Figure 5.5 Change of vertical angle of tool blade from substrate while making dynamic marks.

If a particular face of the tool has been identified from the initial examination, make the first set of test marks using that face. Otherwise, make marks using both faces of the tool and label the test marks with the identification used in the initial examination, and also indicate the direction of movement of the tool. Casts should be made of the test marks. These should be made in the same material as the scene cast, if that is suitable for use on the comparator, otherwise make a replica cast of the scene cast and cast the test marks in a suitable material. Mount the test cast on one comparator stage and the scene cast (or replica cast) on the other, using a suitable mounting material. Make the surfaces of interest as perpendicular as possible to the optic axis and have both directions of movement of the tools in the same orientation. Rotate the stages so that the striations are perpendicular to the dividing line in the comparator eyepiece.

Start with a low magnification and a broad beam of light (if this facility is available) to get both scene and test casts in focus. If the system has par focal lenses then go to the highest magnification and refocus the casts, after which return to the magnification that will be used for the examination. A balance is needed between that required to see the relevant detail and the need to see as much of the mark as possible. It is rarely necessary to go above a total magnification of $\times 50$. Now adjust the lighting if possible/necessary to give a relatively narrow beam of light at a grazing angle of incidence perpendicular to the direction of the striae and which gives good relief to the areas of interest. Use the $x–y$ adjustments of the comparator stages to bring the striae into alignment. In most cases the exact detail will change along the length of the test mark (and potentially in the scene mark as well) so the test mark should be scanned along its length against the scene mark. If no match is found between the test mark made with one side of the tool, compare the test mark from the other side in the same way. If necessary, also look at different points along the scene mark in the same way. If there is more than one scene mark and no link has been found to the first one, consider looking at other marks

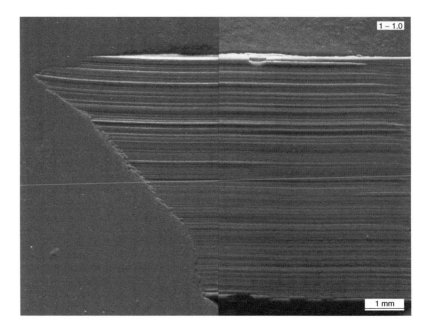

Figure 5.6   Comparison of casts from a striated mark and test pull mark.

in case either detail on the tool has changed or more than one tool has been used. Eventually the image obtained should be similar to that in Figure 5.6.

While images such as this are common in textbooks and forensic science papers, they are far less common in practice. In Figure 5.6 the mark has clear edges, which allows for an easy alignment. In practice, it is worth examining repeat test marks, one against the other, to determine if there is any clearly obvious feature that reliably appears and then look for this in the scene mark. If this feature can be found, then look for confirming striae occurring at the same relative positions to the feature in both marks. For example, there is a wide groove containing finer striae next to a narrow and deep groove about one fifth of the way from the top of the mark as shown in the figure, which could act as such a feature. At this point in the book the emphasis is on the examination, how to evaluate the findings will be covered in the following chapter. Look for the greatest number of corresponding striae, keeping in mind that the narrower the striation the more likely it is that it can change.

The mark in Figure 5.6 illustrates two further points. Firstly, the striae do not exactly correspond over the full width of the mark. This is commonly found and is normally due to the scene mark and the test mark having been made in different materials. These will behave in different ways when subjected to pressure and recover in different ways after the pressure is released, so that the mark will have slightly larger dimensions in one of the materials. Secondly, notice that the striae in the mark on the left are not

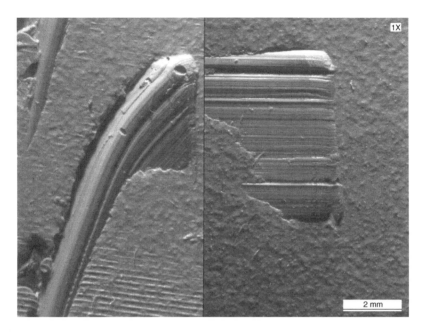

Figure 5.7 Comparison of casts from a foreshortened mark (left) and test mark (right). Note that the test mark has to be rotated to enable alignment of the striations.

exactly perpendicular to the direction of the apparent tip of the tool. It is therefore possible that the tool blade was slightly twisted with respect to the direction of movement of the tool. In this case, the striae appear closer together than in a mark made with the tool blade at right angles to the direction of movement; this effect is sometimes known as 'foreshortening' as we have already discussed in Chapter 4. If this has happened to any great extent in the scene mark, it can be compensated for by rotating the test mark specimen stage so that the striae show a similar foreshortening with regard to the dividing line shown in the objective (Figure 5.7). It is good practice to confirm this by making a further test mark with a similar foreshortening angle to that indicated by the stage rotation. If no great similarity can be seen between the scene and test marks, it is worthwhile rotating the scene mark through 180°, as it is not an easy matter to determine the direction of movement of the tool that made scene mark.

At this point in the examination it may become apparent that a better test mark is needed. The examination should have suggested how the new test mark is to be made, increased pressure, a particular narrow range of vertical angles to the material used for the mark, a different material for the test mark or including foreshortening for example. Unless there is an understanding of how the parameters employed in making the original test mark are to be changed, there is little point in making random test marks in the hope that a better correspondence will be found with the scene mark.

The final stage is to record the degree of correspondence found. This is preferably achieved through photography; modern comparators can be supplied with digital cameras and the images stored on computer or printed out for case notes. It is possible to describe the comparison in words and sketches, but this is more subjective. If described, note the approximate percentage of corresponding striae, any significant disagreement between the scene and test marks and the life-size length/area of comparison being considered.

For cutting marks made by a knife for example, the comparison process is similar to that described above, once suitable test marks have been made and cast. Even if the scene mark is in a small diameter wire, the initial test marks are usually best made by using the whole blade, if possible, to cut through a block of material such as modelling/dental wax rather than trying to make a whole series of cuts in small diameter material. If a specific area is subsequently identified, test marks can then be made in a smaller diameter material to mimic the way the scene mark was made.

5.4.2 Double-bladed cutting tools

In use, a double-bladed cutting tool will leave four cut surfaces, one from each face of the two blades (Figure 5.8). In the initial examination, the blades should have been identified and labelled. Before making the test cut, check to see if there are any indications which parts of the tool blades were used to make the crime cut(s). This is important since, depending on the type and size of tool, each blade can be up to 7 cm or more, making the total length of mark to be examined in the test cuts potentially around 28 cm or more. Label the test cut so that it is clear which side of which blade produced the relevant part of the test mark. Also note the direction that blade is pointing; once the test material is severed these directions are not obvious.

Preparing a test mark does not usually present a problem. The main decision to be made is what material should be used to receive the mark. Traditionally lead is the material of choice. It is readily available and lies in a hardness range that is capable of reproducing striae without causing further damage to the tool. Lead, as supplied, is normally in the form of a sheet and by folding it over it can be made thick enough to 'cut' using a tool with centre-meet blades. As the tool was not intended for use with lead, the folded sheet is rarely severed and, in this case, separating the parts needs to be done carefully to preserve the test mark.

Using lead rod is a better option and it is possible to buy this in different diameters. A single, longitudinal cut is to be preferred over a number of transverse cuts (Figure 5.9). The cut can be made in the rod as supplied or the end of a wider rod can be flattened in a vice. Although this presents the problem of separating the two sides, this is not usually necessary as the test cuts can

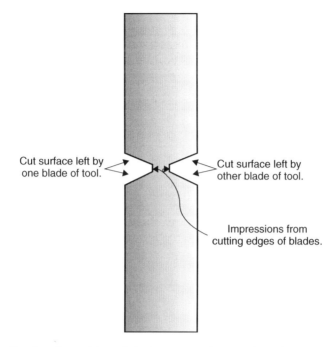

Cut surface left by
one blade of tool.

Cut surface left by
other blade of tool.

Impressions from
cutting edges of blades.

Figure 5.8 Showing the position of the four cut surfaces and two impressions likely to be made by a double-bladed cutting tool.

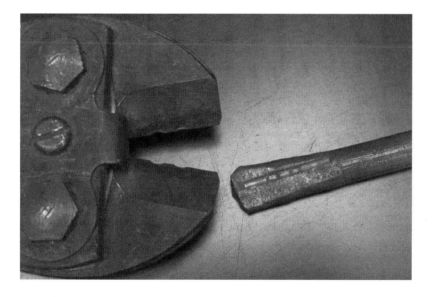

Figure 5.9 Longitudinal test cut made in lead rod, ready for casting.

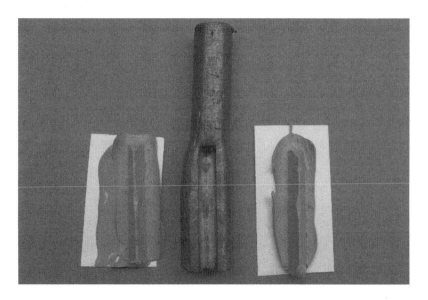

Figure 5.10   Test cut marks cast for detailed comparison.

normally be manipulated under a microscope to look for potentially matching detail without the need to look at individual cut surfaces. It is also possible to use modelling wax or dental wax, which can be bought in the form of bite strips for use in dentistry, or could be melted and cast into rods for test marks. While this is rather soft, it will show the striae. The test cuts and crime cuts (if submitted as the original item) should be cast for detailed comparison (Figure 5.10). While it is possible to work directly from the scene mark and the lead test mark – the lead tarnishes fairly quickly and this, by lowering its reflectivity, makes it easier to light for microscopy – it is better to work with casts.

Mount the scene cast and the test cast on the comparator stages in the same way as for impressed marks; it is possible to mount more than one test cast but practice is needed to get all the casts perpendicular to the optic axis together with good lighting. If you have been able to identify the direction in which the blade tip was pointing in the crime cut, ensure that the casts are all oriented in the same way – that is the blade tip ends are all in the same direction and centre meets are on the same side. The area of interest is normally close to the centre meet. As the blade passes through the material, the part away from the cutting edge tends to 'overwrite' the striae formed by the imperfections present on the edge (Figure 5.11).

As with the sliding marks, decide on a reliably produced and obvious feature present in the scene mark and use a relatively low magnification to scan through the test marks to discover if a similar feature is present in the test marks. If a similar feature can be found, check how many other striae around it also correspond. Although this is a good starting point, sometimes

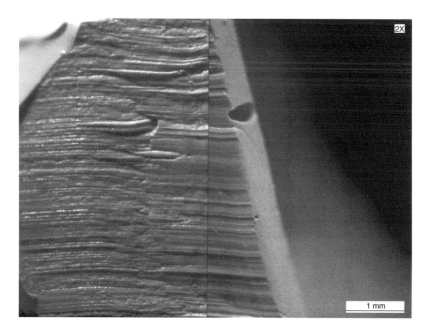

Figure 5.11 Cast of cut mark (left half of image) showing 'overwritten' striations.

there is good detail produced by large imperfections on the face of the blade well away from the cutting edges. This is not modified by the rest of the blade passing over the same area and may be a more reliable area to concentrate on than detail close to the edge itself.

Although marks made by double-bladed cutting tools are being dealt with in this section, remember that the area of best detail may be on the cutting face itself in the form of impressed detail. If the initial examination has shown the presence of good impressed detail in the mark, then that may be a better place to start. The detailed comparison of impressed marks is covered in an earlier section.

5.4.3 Stab marks (in tyres and bones)

Stab marks in tyres combine a variety of types of detail, in part impressed, in part striated and in part deformation of the material receiving the stab. Stab marks in bones can also be considered here as the general principles are similar, but other types of mark in bone (impressed and sawn marks, for example) should be compared following the guidelines given for those particular types of detailed examination once the marks have been cast. What the examiner has on the bench is an object with a hole or a slice in it and they need to see the detail inside the hole. Care must be taken in choosing a casting material to ensure that the hardened cast has the maximum

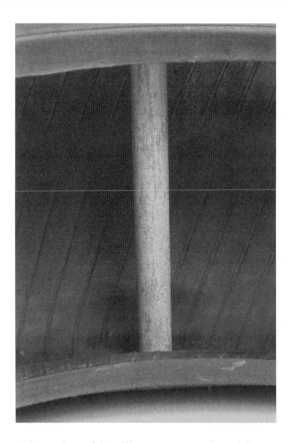

Figure 5.12   Using a piece of dowelling to open a stab mark in a tyre for casting.

mechanical strength so that it can be removed. If the casting material stays in the mark, there is little to nothing that can be done to recover the situation.

For marks in tyres, the two sides of the 'cut' need to be exposed by pushing the tyre from the inside. Stretchers, in the form of simple wooden rods of different lengths can be used to achieve this (Figure 5.12). As well as allowing a visual examination, this also allows the mark to be cast more easily. When the cast has hardened further, open out the mark, which makes the removal of the cast easier. Take time in easing it out and do not use too much force in a direct pull (Figure 5.13). Additionally, the area of tyre around each mark can be cut out (after obtaining any necessary permission to do so) and such pieces can be manipulated more readily. This visual examination and examination of any casts should reveal fine detail in the form of striations (Figure 5.14). If the tyre has been slashed these striations will run parallel to the walls of the tyre (Figure 5.15). For stab marks these go through the tyre wall, although the striations are often curved as the tyre deforms under pressure of the knife point. Very sharp, undamaged blades will show very fine striations. Smooth edged but damaged blades will have coarser detail as

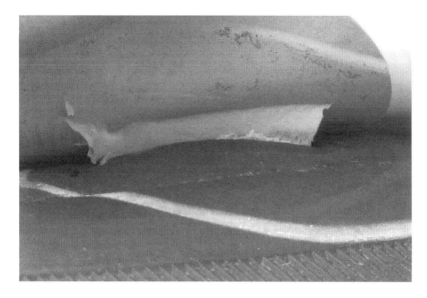

Figure 5.13 Easing casting material out of a tyre stab mark.

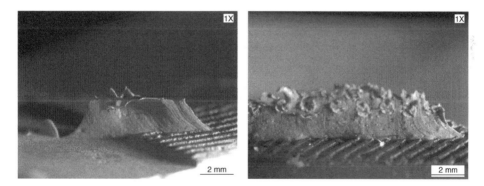

Figure 5.14 Casts of two stab marks, showing distortion and curvature typical of that seen in tyre stabbings.

well as the fine background detail. If a serrated blade has been used this will show as a series of alternating areas of coarse and fine detail (Figure 5.16).

Examination of suspected implements should start with those of a suitable type to leave marks similar to those in the tyre (e.g. there is no relevance in comparing a standard knife against a mark made by a simple pointed object). The implement can be checked for traces of tyre rubber, but many implements used in stabbing tyres do not have such traces and the value of the presence of tyre rubber alone is not very significant. Test marks should then be made in a tyre (in the authors' experience this does not have to be inflated) trying to replicate the action (stabbing or slashing) used in the actual

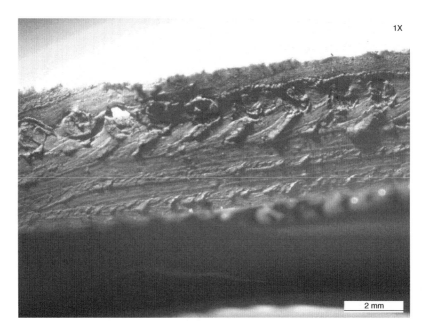

Figure 5.15 Cast of slash mark in a tyre showing striations running along the thickness of the tyre wall, not going through it.

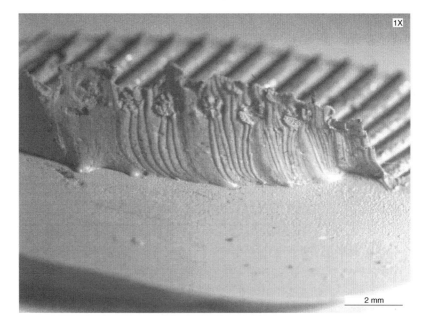

Figure 5.16 Cast of detail in a stab mark made by a serrated blade.

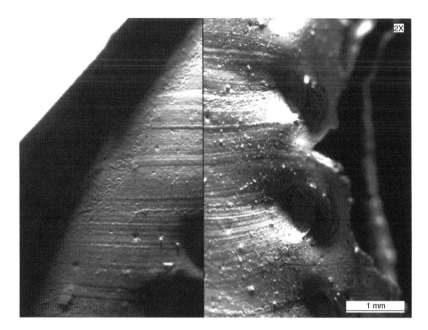

Figure 5.17 Comparison of casts of test stab mark (left) and crime mark (right) showing good corresspondence, but also some distortion.

crime. Once cast, detail in these test marks can then be compared with the crime marks. Often these comparisons show good agreement in the relative disposition of the striations, but there are variations in the exact disposition due to distortions and slight differences in the angle of attack – many marks show striations closer and further apart as they progress through the width of the tyre wall (Figure 5.17).

Post-mortem samples are extremely variable in nature, but ultimately a cast of the mark should be obtained for detailed examination, giving sufficient time for the casting material to develop a good mechanical strength. For most cases of this type, modelling or dental wax is a good material for making test marks, at least as a beginning. Other materials mimicking the mechanical properties of human tissue may be more suitable for marks in cartilage. Dip-Pak™ (a brand of cellulose acetate butyrate) has been used for this purpose (Rao and Hart, 1983), but we understand that it may no longer be available. However, it may be possible to obtain suitable samples of cellulose acetate butyrate from companies such as Evans Coatings, LLC (http://www.evanscoatings.com/) (C. Clow, personal communication, 2012). Other similar materials are available, although the authors cannot recommend any particular one for use for this purpose. In those cases where the tool has a sufficiently characteristic profile, a cast of the relevant part of the tool can be used for direct comparison.

The comparator can be used for the detailed examination and is set up according to whether the impressed detail or the striae are the more important features in the scene mark. In some cases macro photography can be used for the examination, especially when the shape of the mark is the more important aspect of the mark.

It is difficult to express in words how well the scene and test marks correspond for these types of item. The best record is a series of images, as very often it is not possible to capture all the relevant points in one image. It is important for the evaluation to note any significant features that do not correspond and any evidence for the reason why they do not.

5.5   Saw marks

Once the initial comparison has been carried out and the examiner has recovered any suitable trace materials, the ends can be examined in more detail and, if available, compared with the suspect saw(s).

5.5.1   Initial and final cuts

Whatever material the saw marks are in, look especially at initial or final cuts (Figure 5.18). These can contain information relating to the set and spacing of the saw teeth. If material is available from both sides of the cut they should be fitted back together as this could indicate the width of the cut.

The detail in both initial and final cuts is generally similar as it is caused by the final pass of the saw blade over the surface before the saw is removed. The detail is best seen in casts taken from these partial marks, but can also be seen on the original surface.

Figure 5.19 shows initial cuts on a sawn piece of metal rod and a cast taken from it. The cuts have been made by several different saws as can be seen from differences in the widths of the cuts. Most of them contain detail relating to the spacing and set of the saw blades. The one on the extreme right also shows that the blade was in poor condition as the cut is far from sharp and parallel.

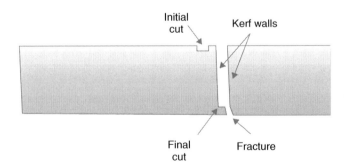

Figure 5.18 Positions of initial and final cuts. See also the photographs of saw marks in Figure 4.24.

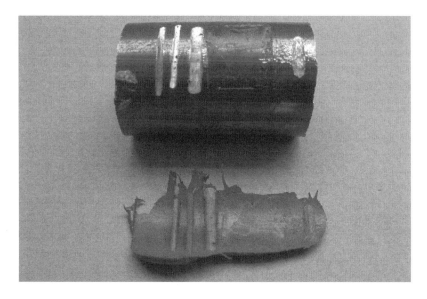

Figure 5.19 Initial cuts on a sawn piece of metal rod and a cast of the cuts.

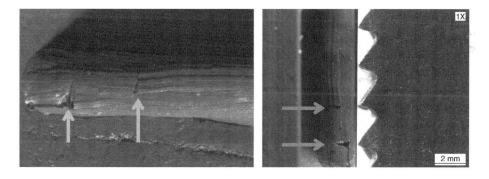

Figure 5.20 Cast teeth impressions in an initial cut (left) compared with a saw blade (right).

Where impressions of teeth are found these should be compared with the suspect saw blade(s) to look at tooth spacing and also to check if the set corresponds (Figure 5.20). Alternatively, they can be checked against blades of known tooth spacing and set to determine the type of blade that was used.

5.5.2 Sawn ends

As well as the partial cuts, the sawn ends may also contain detail that could be linked back to a particular type of saw. This is demonstrated in Figure 5.21. There are usually lines running across the sawn ends (kerf walls), each one representing a single pass of the saw blade. These often run at different

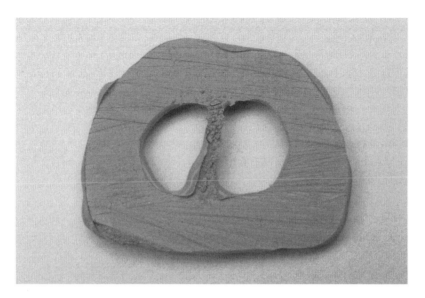

Figure 5.21 Cast of the end of a sawn bone showing lines running across the kerf wall at different angles as the saw moved around.

angles as the saw, or object being sawn, is moved around. The coarseness of these lines can be indicative of the type of saw being used. The finer teeth usually remove less material with each pass of the blade than the coarser ones. Thus, marks made by a 32 tpi blade will be closer together than those made with an 18 tpi blade, which in turn will be closer than those made with a 7 tpi blade. This general trend should also be confirmed by checking the width of the marks, as the finer teeth also tend to be associated with cuts made by narrower blades, although the wavy set may produce a wider kerf than expected from the finer teeth. Occasionally a saw will be used by taking much shorter strokes and this will have the effect of removing less material with each pass, making the lines closer together than might be expected. If a circular saw has been used the lines will be slightly curved. Very occasionally a hacksaw blade may be handheld and this usually means that less material is removed with each pass and in extreme cases the sawn ends can end up being polished by the blade.

As well as checking these marks for coarseness, also look for tooth impressions or waves that can indicate the tooth spacing. This examination must be carried out using oblique lighting, moving the object or cast around as the angle of lighting can affect the detail that can be seen (as shown in Figure 5.22). If any waves have been found these should be compared with either the suspect saw blade(s) or with blades of known tooth spacing, as in Figure 5.23. The sawn ends should also be examined for the presence of scratches caused by teeth slipping across the sawn surface or impressions

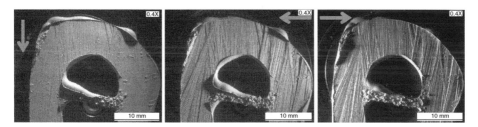

Figure 5.22 Effects of lighting the same marks from different angles, as indicated by the arrows.

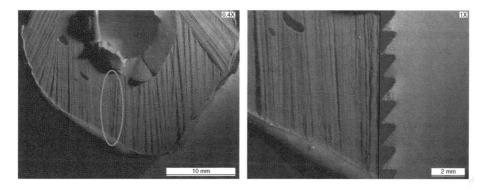

Figure 5.23 Wavy lines (left) and comparison with a saw blade (right).

of teeth that have been pressed into the kerf wall, as in Figure 5.24. These impressions or scratches should then be compared with the suspect saw blade(s) or blades with known tooth spacing. Figure 5.25 shows examples of both of these types of comparison.

5.6 Specialised marks

There are many different types of examination that fall under the broad heading of tool marks, but are not the standard levering or cutting normally associated with forced entry to property or removal of fixed items from premises. A selection of these is given below as examples, but the skilled tool mark examiner should be able to apply the same principles to varied scenarios not covered here.

5.6.1 Alphanumeric punches

The comparisons for this type of examination are essentially the same as for basic impressed marks. The main difficulties encountered relate to how the implements that make the marks are made.

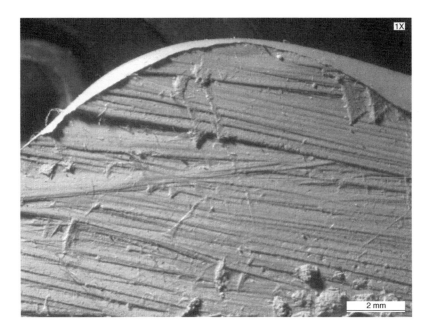

Figure 5.24   Cast impressions of teeth in the kerf wall.

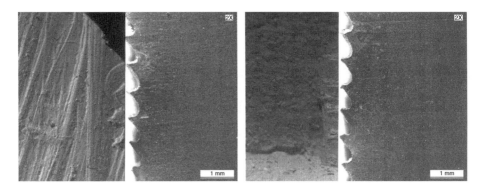

Figure 5.25   Comparisons of casts of teeth impressions (left) and scratches (right) on kerf wall with suspect saw blade.

   Number punches are produced in bulk. The character is pressed onto the end of a piece of stock steel and these are then finished off and may be plated. Many punches may have the characters formed by using the same die and thus much of the detail on a new punch will relate to the production die used and any imperfections in it. However, owing to the nature of use of such tools, microscopic damage and chipped plating will be rapidly acquired. It is necessary for the examiner to be able to determine what is class detail and what is unique. Weimar *et al.* (2010) consider detail that is present on new punches.

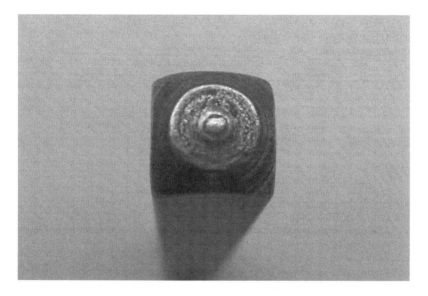

Figure 5.26 End of blank punch before the character is imparted onto it.

To make a number punch the relevant character is engraved onto each face of a hardened steel cube (the 'hob' that is used to form the characters on the final stamp). This gives the basic shape and form of the character and all six faces will show the same basic detail. Depending on the method of engraving, however, there will be differences in the fine detail produced in the characters on the different faces of the hob. A piece of stock steel is cut to the length of the punch and is roughly milled and ground to shape (Figure 5.26). One end of this is then forced against one face of the hob to impress the character onto the end of the punch. Much of the fine detail, as well as the general shape and form of the character, will be imparted at this stage. To complete the punch, the end will be ground to give the circular or ovoid background to the character and details will be punched onto the side of the shank (Figure 5.27). The punch will then normally be plated to give its final appearance (Figure 5.28). Over a period of time more than one hob will be used to make punches of the same style, giving rise to more variations in sub-class characteristics. It should be borne in mind that a set of punches would be put together by combining one of each of the characters from stocks that have been made previously and that different sets are likely to contain a mixture of punches made using different hobs. Thus, if the sub-class details can be discerned, the combination of punches would have a degree of significance. With use the hobs would become damaged and this damage, although still not unique to a particular punch, would increase the significance of any match that was found. A detailed description of the manufacturing and detail on alphanumeric punches is given in a paper by Van Dijk (1985).

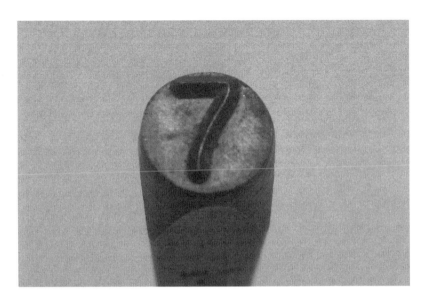

Figure 5.27   Unplated punch with the number embossed onto the end, shaped by grinding the edges.

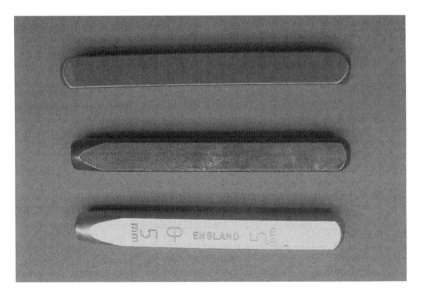

Figure 5.28   Three stages of producing a number punch from blank (top), through unplated punch with the number embossed onto the end that has now been shaped by grinding the edges (middle) to the finished plated punch (bottom).

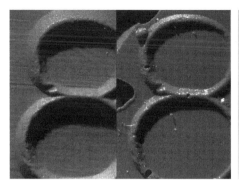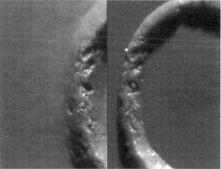

Figure 5.29 Two examples of detail in casts of test marks made with number punches compared with casts of crime marks.

Card embossing machines also utilise punches to produce the characters onto plastic cards. Unlike the number punches just described, card embossing machines have two parts that work in unison. While these punches can be made in similar ways to number punches, they are more likely to be cast in metal from masters, thus ensuring that the same detail is reproduced on many machines. It is important for the examiner to be satisfied that any detail reproduced on cards is caused by damage to the punches that has been acquired during manufacture or use. Often detail is present not only from the character part of the punches, but also at least part of the surrounding area of the punch makes contact, leaving its own characteristics on the card.

For both types of examination, having determined that the punches or embossing machine supplied have characters of the correct size and shape, test marks should be made using the relevant characters. These test marks can then be compared with casts of the crime marks, looking at the specific shapes of individual characters to ensure there are no significant differences. If the characters are correct, then look for evidence of damage either on the characters themselves or on surrounding areas if those have come into contact with the item that has been embossed, particularly on credit cards. Figure 5.29 shows two examples of comparisons of detail on number punches.

5.6.2 Drill marks

Most drill marks comprise simply the final, complete hole through the surface being drilled. Even if there is fine detail around the circumference of the hole, it is unlikely that this type of mark would give more information than the diameter of the drill bit used. This would not be highly significant. What is required is material where marks have been left by the cutting end of the bit as it rotated during the drilling process. This could be in the form of either incomplete marks or swarf produced by the drilling process (usually found

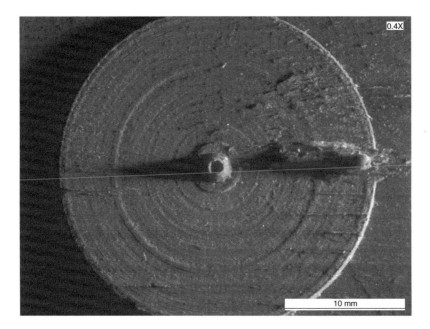

Figure 5.30   Cast of an incomplete drill mark, showing striation detail.

below the drilled area) (Figure 5.30). Even when no fine detail is present, such marks could show the general profile of the drill tip as well as the diameter.

Drill bits are worn down through use and the profile will change. This is normally a slow process, but when a very hard object is being drilled this can happen very rapidly. In some circumstances, if the object being drilled is a mixture of hard and soft material, the drill bit may be completely re-profiled. In these circumstances finding a match of the profile would be highly significant, even in the absence of fine characteristic detail (which would change rapidly with subsequent use) (Figure 5.31). Ideally, there will be a series of concentric striations on the surface that is being drilled. These striations are produced by the cutting edges at the very tip of the bit acting like miniature chisels and can potentially be linked back to test marks made with the drill bit in the same way as other marks containing striations. The test marks should be made by twisting the bit (either by hand or fitted in the drill) against lead or a modelling/dental wax sheet and the resultant marks should be cast.

5.6.3   Slide hammers

In most cases where a slide hammer, as described in Chapter 3, has been used, it will be necessary to link the screw back to any marks in a lock barrel found at the scene. The first problem is visualising the relevant detail, which will be inside the keyway of the lock barrel. This could be done by dismantling

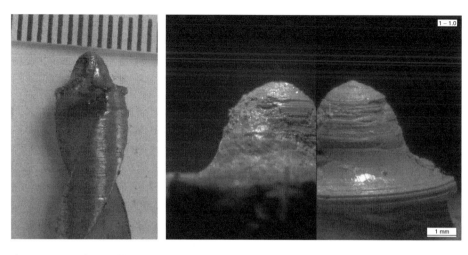

Figure 5.31   The profile of a drill bit (left) has been heavily modified by drilling through a hardened material; a comparison photograph of partial drill mark casts (right) shows a good correspondence in the shapes of a mark from the scene and a test mark made using this drill bit.

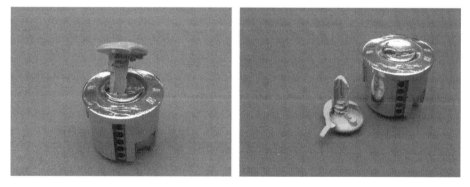

Figure 5.32   Removing casting material from the keyway (left) and the cast of the keyway, showing screw detail (right).

the lock, but there is no guarantee that all of the detail could be retrieved in exactly the same relative positions as the components could move around. The most effective way is to use a highly fluid, slow curing silicone rubber compound. Such materials need to be left to cure for 24 hours, but they should flow into the relevant areas of the keyway. The cast needs to be removed carefully and slowly, and it should have replicated as much of the detail as possible (Figure 5.32).

Once removed, the cast should be examined for detail left by the screw responsible. At the very least it should show the thread pitch and the diameter of the screw. These vary with different types and sizes of screw and should be compared with not only the screw still fitted to the slide hammer, but also with any loose screws found associated with the suspect. At this stage this can be done by mounting the cast from the lock barrel on the comparator along with the actual screw, as no fine detail is involved. There may also be damage to the screw that is replicated in the mark left by the forced impact of the screw in the keyway in the form of an impression. If any fine detail is noted on the cast from the barrel, when examining under a bench microscope using oblique directional lighting, the screw should be examined for any areas bearing similar detail. A replica cast should then be made of any such areas. Alternatively, a suitable medium such as lead or a modelling/dental wax sheet can be pressed against the relevant area to make a test mark, which should then be cast for a detailed comparison.

5.6.4   Pipe cutters

Reference was made earlier in Chapter 4 to pipe cutters. The action of pipe cutters is different from that of other cutting tools. Rather than slicing through an object leaving marks running across the cut end, pipe cutters are fitted around a pipe or other cylindrical object that is to be cut and the tool is rotated around the circumference. A simple pipe cutter comprises a single rotating cutting disc that goes on one side of the pipe and rollers that go onto the opposite side. Other pipe cutters are designed for cutting larger diameter tubes (of similar diameter to those on vehicle exhaust systems) and have a series of rotating cutting discs fitted onto a chain, which is wrapped around the tubing.

For both types the cutter is rotated around the object being cut and the discs press into the surface, rotating as they go, getting deeper with each rotation, until the pipe is severed. This results in a series of almost concentric striations around the cut surface. These often show no useful characteristic detail. Of much more use are any partial cuts around the outside of the pipe before the cutter has started to go through the material, in much the same way as initial cuts in saw mark cases. If the cutting disc has damage around the circumference, especially in the form of notches, these will leave characteristic detail in these initial cuts.

The marks should be cast and the relative positions, sizes and shapes of these imperfections can be compared with those in casts of partial test cuts made using the suspected pipe cutter in similar diameter material. The rollers do not play an active part in cutting through the pipe, but they rotate around the outer surface. Good condition rollers just leave a slightly burnished area around either side of the cut, but if there is any damage or burring to the edge of the roller this can be impressed into the surface and can be as characteristic as detail on the disc. As this detail will also appear to the side of a complete cut, as well as partial cuts, this may be a means of linking a pipe cutter to a completely severed object where there are no partial cuts.

5.7 Other considerations

5.7.1 Test marks made *in situ*

The industrial guillotine is used here as an example of the type of heavy machinery where comparisons involve using controls made *in situ* because it was impossible to remove and transport it to the laboratory. The tool mark examiner will need to be aware of how the equipment is used and to ensure that there is sufficient control material to cover the full extent of the cutting blade and to show potential variations in detail produced when the same area is used on different occasions. This can be achieved by comparing different pieces of the test material to see how they relate to each other. In this example several pieces of lead have been cut by the guillotine, and Figure 5.33 shows how the three pieces overlap with the same features appearing in different positions on them, to cover a wider area of the cutting surface. Without access to the actual machinery, the examiner will also have to evaluate the detail observed to determine if it is characteristic and not class detail that would have been imparted to many different machines during manufacture.

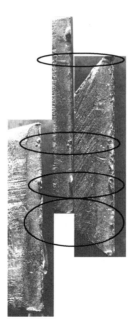

Figure 5.33   Three industrial guillotine marks, aligned to show corresponding detail.

5.7.2   Amount of detail required for comparison

It is often thought that the larger the area of mark, the better it is for comparison with a tool. This can be a mistake, as it is not the area of mark that is important in carrying out a tool mark comparison, but the amount of characteristic detail that is present within the mark. A large area of mark may not even contain enough detail to identify reliably the size and shape of tool used if it comprises multiple overlapping impressions in a rough and degraded surface. On the other hand, a mark no larger than the size of a pinhead (or even smaller), when made in a smooth surface that takes very good fine detail, can contain more than sufficient characteristic features, even though it is not possible to determine the type of tool responsible. One example shown in Figure 5.34 is a very small mark (of pinhead size) made in metal beading by the very corner of a screwdriver blade. This is typical of the sort of mark that may be made when beading is removed from a glazed window or door panel by inserting a tool between the beading and the fixed frame and twisting. A microscopic examination of the original item and a cast made from it will reveal the presence of potentially characteristic detail in the form of grinding and damage from the surface of the tool.

5.7.3   Use of a scanning electron microscope (SEM)

The vast majority of comparisons are carried out using optical microscopy. As discussed elsewhere, this works well, even for small areas of mark providing the detail can be imaged by conventional light optics.

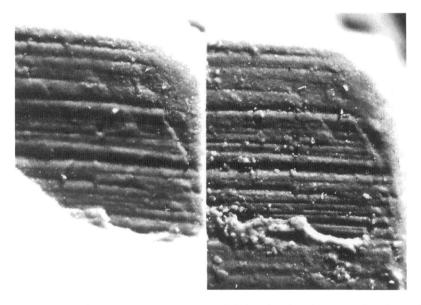

Figure 5.34   Cast of a very small tip corner mark (of pinhead size) compared with a replica cast of the suspect tool.

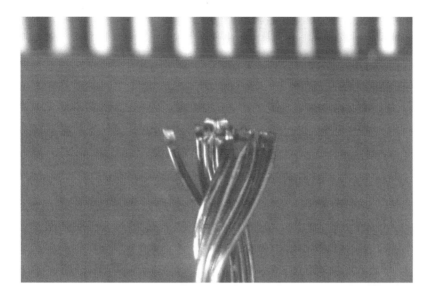

Figure 5.35 The cut end of a braided wire, showing tool marks on the ends of some strands.

This is not, however, the lower limit of being able to carry out tool mark comparisons. Mention was made in Chapter 3 of braided cables being cut (Figure 5.35). These may not contain any fine detail imparted by the tool, but very occasionally there can be impressions of detail left on individual strands of wire within the cable. While this may be visible and its presence noted under an optical microscope, the depth of field may not be sufficient to resolve and readily compare that detail under an optical comparator. Another example relates to staples. These are normally used in a stapler, which has a plunger (usually in the form of a simple metal strip) (Figure 5.36) that is pressed against the top of the staple to push it through the material to be stapled together and in the same operation to bend over the points of the staple. In this instance, the end of the plunger can be considered as being a tool and can potentially leave characteristic impressed (and even sliding) marks on the upper surface of the staples. As with braided cable, the area of the mark is very small and the detail correspondingly fine, so it would be difficult to use optical microscopy for the examination. Test marks in this type of case would involve using the stapler on a series of staples, which could allow variations between the detail produced on them to be assessed.

For both the braided cable and stapler examples, if the initial examination has shown the presence of small areas of interest containing very fine detail (in crime and test samples) that could not be satisfactorily resolved using optical microscopy, all is not lost. If the case warrants a more detailed comparison and an SEM is available for use, and it is possible to introduce the crime and test materials into the equipment, detail much finer than that resolvable under an optical microscope can be visualised and compared. Because the

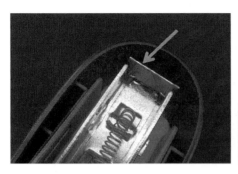
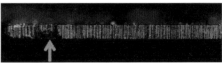

Figure 5.36 A stapler, with plunger (left) and an SEM photograph of half of the ground leading edge of the plunger, with an area of damage (right).

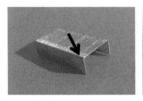
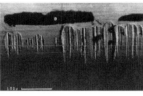
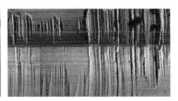

Figure 5.37 Typical staples with 'top bar' indicated by arrow (left); dynamic grinding detail on the top bar of a staple from the scene was photographed using a scanning electron microscope (middle) and compared with a photograph of a test mark made with the plunger of the suspect stapler (right – top shows crime mark, bottom shows test mark).

detail is so fine and potentially variable, SEM photographs can be taken of the end of the wire strand and the relevant area of a series of test marks made by the suspected cutters. Likewise, a series of SEM photographs could be taken along the surface of crime and test staples. The resultant photographs can then be compared side by side, looking at the fine characteristic detail that is present (Figure 5.37).

References

Rao, V.J. and Hart, R. (1983) Tool mark determination in cartilage of stabbing victim. *Journal of Forensic Sciences*, **28** (3), 794–799.

Van Dijk, T.M. (1985) Steel marking Stamps. Their individuality at the time of manufacture. *Journal of the Forensic Science Society*, **25** (4), 243–253.

Weimar, B., Balzer, J. and Weber, M. (2010) The identifying characteristics of new marking stamps. *The Information Bulletin for Shoeprint/Toolmark Examiners*, **16** (1), 17–45.

6

Interpretation and Evaluation

6.1 Introduction

In order to provide a conclusion to an examination, the findings will need to be interpreted and evaluated. Generally, in this chapter we will mean 'interpretation' to be an explanation of what you have observed and 'evaluation' to be the weighing up of what the interpretation findings mean with respect to prosecution and defence cases. These two processes are intrinsically linked and in some cases are carried out almost simultaneously in the expert's mind as the comparison progresses. There have been numerous good publications in the scientific literature covering the various aspects of interpretation and evaluation relating to this field: the principles of case assessment, how tools are produced and whether their features are class, sub-class or individual, statistical approaches to evaluation, to name but a few. A sample of such literature is given in this book in the references we have used for the various chapters. However, any library database or Internet search would give more examples if further research were necessary on specific topics. In this chapter we will try to summarise what we feel is best practice.

6.1.1 Interpretation

As previously discussed in Chapter 1, at a fundamental level, a tool mark comparison can be considered to be a comparison of the 'unknown' or 'questioned' material (marks recovered from the crime scene) with the 'known' (a suspect, control or reference item, which is usually a tool of some type). The aim of the comparison process is therefore to determine what features and detail of the 'unknown' correspond to, or differ from, those on the 'known'.

The Forensic Examination and Interpretation of Tool Marks, First Edition.
David Baldwin, John Birkett, Owen Facey and Gilleon Rabey.
© 2013 John Wiley & Sons, Ltd. Published 2013 by John Wiley & Sons, Ltd.

If features are present in a mark that match features on a tool's surface or those made by it in a test mark, it will be necessary to explain what the features are and what process, random or otherwise, caused them to be there. If they differ, it will be necessary to consider whether the differences are significant (and therefore the tool can be discounted) or if there is a reasonable and logical explanation that may explain the difference.

This interpretation of matching and non-matching features is vital to enable the court reporting scientist to build up a picture of the overall evidential significance of the findings in their evaluation. This also emphasises the necessity of the practitioner to have good background knowledge of manufacturing processes and also an awareness of how wear and tear can affect a tool's surface over time.

When an expert is carrying out a marks' comparison, considerations will include the following.

- The definition and quality of any detail in a mark, depending on the substrate, pressure used to make the mark and so on.

- The amount and character of the detail present on the suspect tool and whether or not you would expect to find it reproduced in a mark. For example, if there is no detail then other tools with the same class features could potentially produce the same marks.

- The amount and character of the detail present in the mark and how well it corresponds (or not) to features on the tool.

- If features have been produced in a way that would mean they could be present on more than one tool or not be distinguishable between tools produced in a similar way. For example, pressed lines, milling, broaching and so on.

- If features have been randomly acquired and are therefore considered to be unique, i.e. they would not be found on any other tool. For example, grinding or damage detail.

- How various external factors can affect the detail seen in crime scene marks and on the surface of a control item (and therefore could contribute to any apparent differences between them). Factors that could affect the detail seen could include the type of substrate, the activity, angle and pressure that was used, extraneous particles trapped in between the instrument and substrate, the condition of the item producing the marks and also the recovery and packaging of the marks. Factors that may affect features on the control item, meaning that it is not in the exact same condition as when the marks were made, could include its subsequent use, general wear and tear, damage, corrosion and so on.

6.1.2 Evaluation

It is the evaluation process that will enable the court reporting scientist to make an unbiased judgement on the evidence as a whole. To reiterate the concepts from Chapter 1, a forensic practitioner has a duty to the court to provide evidence (Association of Forensic Science Providers, *Standards for the Formulation of Evaluative Forensic Science Expert Opinion*, 2009), which is:

- logical

- transparent

- balanced

- robust.

In order to be all of these things, practitioners have to make it explicit exactly what they have done and by which method, what features have been considered and why, what allowances have been made and why and, finally and importantly, by clearly laying out a prosecution *and* a defence view against which to consider the findings. These views will undoubtedly be opposing and, in tool mark examinations, more often than not address the potential source of the mark(s). The prosecution view that 'the submitted tool made the scene mark' is not difficult to formulate.

However, it is unlikely that a practitioner for the prosecution would be provided with any formulated defence argument at the outset and therefore it is reasonable to construct one, provided it will help the court to understand the weight of the findings. As the views will be opposing, it may seem reasonable to suggest the opposite, 'this tool did not make the mark', as the defence alternative. However, this is not particularly helpful or logical in this context, as this would leave the defence with a question of 'Well what other tool or how many other tools could have?' Therefore, we would not recommend proposing this as a defence view.

Another defence alternative that could be proposed is, since in their view the submitted tool was not involved, 'another similar tool made the mark'. However, we do not believe that this gives the court sufficient information about how many other tools could have made the mark or signifies the true weight of the evidence (as seemingly another similar tool would give the same level of correspondence as the tool in question, effectively neutralising the weight of the evidence). Nevertheless, there are instances when the practitioner just does not have any idea of the significance of the findings and so can only address this sort of alternative, although we would not recommend this as routine practice.

The method which we would strongly advocate as best practice, is to consider the findings given the prosecution view that 'this tool made the mark', allowing for limitations of the comparison such as substrate, quality, definition and so on, against the defence view of 'some other tool made the mark'. This latter alternative allows the practitioner to assess how likely the findings are if the mark was made by another unknown tool, picked at random from a general population of tools.

The reader may already be aware of Bayes' Theorem, where exclusive propositions such as these can be evaluated, one against the other. The situation is similar here, but at this time there is no accepted way of deriving the probabilities required for using this method in marks' evaluation. While the theorem gives a logical basis for evaluating the results, it cannot be used to provide a numerical result, otherwise known as the 'likelihood ratio[1]'. This is because there is a lack of readily available, reliable data concerning the commonality of tools or features on tools with which to inform these probabilities. Instead a practitioner may express their subjective opinion on the matter, using their knowledge and experience. We would be happy that good practice has been demonstrated, provided the two opposing views outlined above were made explicit and considered in the evaluation of any source level tool marks' comparison. We consider that this is a robust and scientific approach (Biedermann *et al.*, 2012).

The assessment is based on the detail (or lack of detail) that the mark shows, of how common or rare that detail is considered to be and whether fewer or more other tools in that general population could correspond to the same extent as a result. Effectively, as the number of other tools in this general population that could also have been responsible gets smaller, the rarer the detail shown in the mark is considered to be, going from: all tools, to the type of tool that could be responsible for that type of mark (e.g. levering or cutting tools as relevant), to the specific type of tool (e.g. screwdriver or case opener), to those that share the same general shape and size, to those that were manufactured in a similar way or using the same equipment, to those that were all of the above and have the same characteristic features of damage and wear.

---

[1] The likelihood ratio is the ratio of the probability of the findings given the prosecution view and background information (the numerator) over the probability of the findings given the defence view and background information (the denominator) (Aitken, 1995).

With the exception of those cases where the questioned mark is of such limited quality that any tool potentially could have made it, this still leaves a proportion of tools in the general population considered that would differ from the questioned mark (up to the point where all other tools would differ). For example, given a scene mark that has obviously been made by a 9 mm screwdriver, in a general population of other 9 mm screwdrivers some may differ on the basis that they had different shaped tip corners or other such feature that would differentiate them, depending on what other detail the mark showed.

6.1.3   Interpretation and evaluation

In any tool mark examination, a logical thought process should develop to incorporate both interpretation and evaluation, such as:

- *'The shape of the mark differs from the shape of the tool. This is a significant difference, which can only be explained by the submitted tool not being responsible.'*
  This sort of conclusive result may also be known as an 'elimination' or an 'exclusion'.

- *'This mark corresponds in shape and size to the blade of this tool. Detail in this mark corresponds to grinding and damage on the tool's surface. These features are acquired randomly and I would not expect them to be repeated on another tool. Therefore, since there is sufficient detail present of this kind, I feel that this level of correspondence would not be possible with another tool. Therefore it is my expert opinion that this tool made the mark.'*
  This type of conclusive link or 'identification' is not a scientific one, but is expressed as the expert's *opinion* based on their experience, knowledge and belief that there are sufficient corresponding unique features that have been randomly acquired and therefore would not be repeated on any other tool. Practitioners using a purely probabilistic approach would not give such an opinion, but would instead use the highest level on their 'scale of support', which we shall begin to explain subsequently. This gives leeway for the view that as all other tools have not been examined, there may be one in existence that shows the same features, however small this possibility. In terms of probabilistic evaluation, a conclusive link is the equivalent of saying the probability of finding this degree of correspondence with another tool is zero. In other words, it is not a conceivable option. It is not our contention that practitioners who are comfortable with reporting conclusive links should stop, but it should be recognised that they are taking what some may consider to be a 'leap of faith' (Stoney, 1991). In this chapter, we will discuss using a combination of these approaches.

- *'This tip corner mark corresponds in shape to this screwdriver. There is no other detail shown in the mark, which may be due to it having been made in painted, splintered wood. Therefore, this tool could have made the mark; however, there may be another screwdriver or other levering tool with this shape of tip corner in existence that could also have made the mark. Given the limited area of mark and lack of detail, I consider that there are many tools, of all different sizes, that could have left such a mark. However, there is still a small chance that a tool picked at random could show some differences, for example, a screwdriver or other levering tool with a differently shaped tip corner (for whatever reason), and therefore the findings are slightly more likely given the prosecution view than the defence view.'*

Where it cannot be ruled out that another tool was responsible (as above), this leads to an expression of a 'level of support' for a particular view, based on a predetermined 'scale of support'. This may also be thought of as providing a level of 'corroborative' evidence to the court. A level of support in tool marks will usually address the prosecution view, as those tools exhibiting differences from scene marks should, under the best circumstances, have already been eliminated. However, there may be occasions where a level of support is expressed for the defence view. We will develop one scale of support in Section 6.2; however, there are other scales in existence.

It should be noted at this point that the results of the majority of tool mark examinations that the authors' have worked on have either been conclusive eliminations or identifications or, given huge limitations of the mark, it has not been possible to rule out the submitted or any other tool from being responsible. This result is termed an 'inconclusive' result, where *no support* is offered either way. It is not particularly common to get results in between that offer a level of support, unless the practitioner is working from a purely probabilistic point of view.

This re-emphasises the necessity for good police work in submitting suitable items for comparison, of asking the right questions at the beginning of an examination and understanding as much as possible of the circumstances around the incident that gave rise to the mark. Of utmost importance is using the right casting material initially (or preferably having original items bearing the marks submitted whenever possible rather than casts) to replicate and record the detail of a mark at its finest level, as well as having the best equipment available to show any very fine detail in a mark at a high resolution. This leads to the strongest results, which in our view, are easiest to understand and therefore most helpful to the court.

6.1.4   Scene-to-scene linking

Less frequently, the court reporting scientist will be asked to help the investigating officer by giving an opinion concerning the possibility of linking offences by comparing tool marks recovered from different scenes. In this case, the question is often 'Did the same tool make these different crime scene marks?' Usually, one of the crime scene marks is used as a 'control mark' and the others compared with it. Questions asking only for information regarding the type of tool used will not be considered here.

6.2   Considerations as the laboratory examination progresses

6.2.1   Eliminations and inconclusive evidence

The basis for evaluation should be considered from the very start of an examination by having a question that is being asked by the submitting authority clearly formulated. The commonest form is along the lines of 'Did the submitted tool make the crime mark?' As we have already discussed, to prevent any evaluation from becoming unbalanced by considering just one side of the argument, the alternative question 'Did some other tool make the mark?' should also be present in the practitioner's mind. Factors that a marks' practitioner is primarily concerned with are class, sub-class and unique features, already discussed in other chapters of this book.

The preliminary stages of the interpretation and evaluation are taken in the initial examination at the bench. The emphasis is on noting if there are significant differences between the scene mark and the tool such that the tool can be eliminated from having made the mark. Care should be taken to ensure at this early stage that any apparent differences are indeed significant and could not be accounted for by the way in which the mark was made. For example, if the mark appears to be of a different width from the tool, are you certain that it is a single mark and not two overlapping marks showing opposing edges of the tool? In which case, the width in the mark would not necessarily reflect the width of the tool. Or, can you be certain that only one tool has been used at the scene? There may be detail present that allows one area of mark to be eliminated, but another less defined area could be from the tool being examined.

If significant differences can be found then clearly some other tool was responsible for the making the mark and the suspect tool can be eliminated from the enquiry. If the question has not been asked already by this stage, it may be worth investigating whether other tools have been seized in the case.

If the mark has no clear detail, is of limited extent/quality or too poor to give a useful result, for example it may be an indistinct mark bearing a couple of uncharacteristic striae or shows a straight edge only, bearing no other detail, then it may be the practitioner's view that there is no point in continuing the examination. The evidence is effectively inconclusive, that is, there is insufficient support for either of the views that this tool or another one was responsible.

If, after the initial examination, the tool cannot be eliminated and there is sufficient cause to proceed, the examination should become more detailed, involving casting techniques, making test marks and use of a comparator as appropriate. These examinations will generally be those where it is considered that there is either a level of correspondence between the mark and tool (and further work is necessary to demonstrate and record this prior to reaching a formal conclusion), or further work is required to establish whether there is a level of agreement or not.

For sliding marks, comparison of the striation detail can only be done by preparing suitable test marks using the tool. Striations left by imperfections on the tool can be compared with the scene marks. For impressed marks, the comparison will have been carried out using either suitable test marks or by making a replica cast of the tool. The factors being considered in impressed marks include wear (such as rounded tip corners) and grinding detail, irregular surface texture resulting from manufacture or corrosion and also damage features, such as notches, scratches, dents, burrs and gouges.

6.2.2   Identifications and levels of support

Any comparison is limited by the amount and quality of detail present in the mark. However, in general, the more detail that is present as we move through comparisons of class and sub-class features to individual characteristics, the more the evidential value will increase. Obviously at stronger levels of evidence, the less significant features also need to correspond. For example, if a mark shows an area of characteristic detail, such as irregular grinding, then that detail needs to be in the correct position in relation to the tip and edge of the tool.

Under the best circumstances, a clearly defined mark with sufficient characteristic detail can give a conclusive link to the right tool, provided the expert is comfortable with reporting results in this absolute way. If they are not, preferring a purely probabilistic approach, then a term such as *very strong* support could be used, meaning that there may be at least one other tool or very few other tools in existence that could also have made the mark (but even so, the probability of the findings given another tool is vanishingly small).

These sorts of cases can be quick to resolve, because given comparisons with detail equivalent to that shown in Figures 6.1 and 6.2, the interpretation

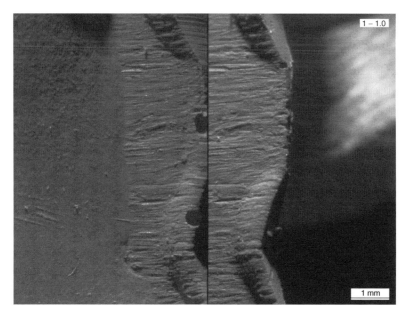

Figure 6.1 Cast of an impressed mark (left), showing excellent correspondence of the characteristic outline of the blade profile, including notches and burring, grinding, other damage and irregularities, to a replica cast of the suspect tool blade (right).

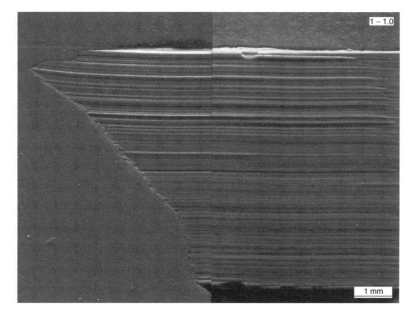

Figure 6.2 Cast of a striated mark (left), showing excellent correspondence of fine and coarse striations to a cast of a test pull mark made with the suspect tool tip (right). Slight misalignment of the individual striations as shown is not uncommon in comparisons of this type. These differences may be due to slight twisting of the tool responsible as it made the mark and also that the crime and test marks were made in different substrates.

is clear; there is an excellent level of correspondence between the questioned mark and representation of the tool. It also needs to be said that comparisons such as this, where it is necessary to look quite hard for apparent discrepancies, are not uncommon. Often the more difficult and time consuming aspect comes not in the comparison of features but in obtaining the best and most appropriate representation of the tool, either as a recast or a test mark. Preliminary test marks may be needed to locate the relevant part of the tool for comparison with the mark, together with how the mark was produced by the tool responsible.

We believe that the illustrated figures speak for themselves in describing what is meant by 'sufficient characteristic detail' and clear and convincing arguments as to why these comparisons lead to the opinion that they were undoubtedly made by the questioned tool would not be difficult to explain or be understood in court. Typically, the arguments fall into two types, the theoretical and the practical, based on experience. The theoretical notes that finding the same random set of characteristic features on another tool is statistically unlikely and, as the number of features increase, verges on the highly improbable. The practical notes that only one orientation of the tool produces a matching test mark. Further, when multiple tools have been examined, the test marks do not match each other. Nor is there any recognised work that has shown significant random features matching in tools.

However, some marks contain less detail than this. Since this area of evidence is highly subjective, different experts will have different views of what level of matching detail is sufficient to give a conclusive result, particularly when the evidence is less clear than the examples shown. There are no hard and fast rules. Suffice to say that if individual characteristics confer uniqueness to a tool's surface, the practitioner must rely on their training and experience to assess how characteristic individual features are and how characteristic the detail is in total.

However, it does not follow that a small area of mark would be less characteristic than a large area of mark. Figure 6.3 shows an area of mark on the top bar of a staple, which is less than half a millimetre wide, taken by a scanning electron microscope. This dynamic mark was produced by grinding detail on the bottom edge of the plunger of a stapler (see Chapter 5 for more details). Even a fraction of this mark could be said to be unique. This again highlights the necessity to be using the correct casting materials, equipment and techniques in order to resolve any fine detail and obtain the best results. Often, this can be done without the use of a scanning electron microscope, but this example shows what is possible. It is not the size of the mark that matters but the quality of the detail present and how it is best recorded and visualised.

Sometimes, a comparison will show a good level of overall agreement, but there may be limitations or some differences in the detail. Limitations could include poor definition due to the substrate and the way that the mark was

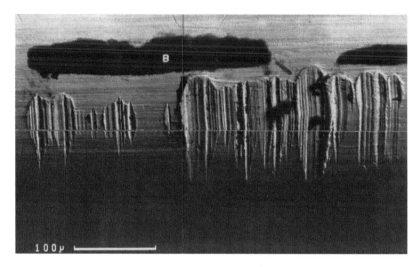

Figure 6.3 Dynamic grinding detail on the top bar of a staple, that has been produced by grinding on the bottom edge of the plunger of a stapler. The area of mark shown is less than half a millimetre wide.

made. Differences may have reasonable explanations, such as the tool being damaged after the mark was made or that the crime and test marks were made in different substrates. In these instances, it may not be possible to say without doubt that the tool made the mark and leaves open the possibility that a small number of other tools could have. The result must be downgraded to a *strong* level of support, assuming that making further test marks does not improve the level of agreement. This level of support would typically be used for impressed marks where there is only an indication of or limited area of corresponding characteristic detail. On occasion 'very strong support' could be used, depending on the amount and clarity of the detail.

For striated marks, it may be that only a proportion of characteristic striations correspond. The number of other tools that could make marks showing the same detail will be small, so there is still a good chance that one picked at random from the general population considered would *not* correspond to the mark to the same extent as the suspect tool. Therefore, the results are much more likely given the prosecution view. In the authors' experience, however, few comparisons fall into this category, because usually the majority of conclusions fall into the categories of elimination, identification (or very strong) or inconclusive, with a few at a low level, such as limited/moderate support.

Starting at the lower end of the scale now, where comparisons involve class features only, with no sub-class or characteristic features, considerations will revolve around the parameters of tool type and general shape and size (where these can be confirmed). This could either be indicated by an impressed mark or the width of a dynamic mark with little other detail. If we go back to the

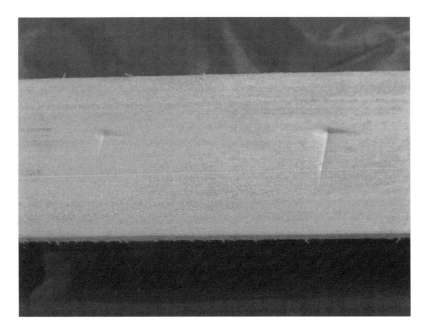

Figure 6.4   Tip corner marks in wood, without any fine detail, that might offer a limited level of support, given that a large number of levering tools of different sizes could have made them.

example given earlier, where the mark contained only a tip corner, which could be said to have been made by a large number of screwdrivers or other levering tools with a similarly shaped tip corner, then there is only a *limited* level of support for the submitted tool having made the mark (Figure 6.4). Whilst this may represent a large number of levering tools, there is still a small chance that one picked at random would differ, for example, screwdrivers or other levering tools with a differently shaped tip corner. Therefore, the results are slightly more likely given the prosecution view.

However, if the mark now showed the shape and size of the screwdriver responsible, this would reduce the number of other screwdrivers that could have been responsible. Although if the size was considered to be a more common one, for example, 9 mm, then a conservative estimate would be that this could still be a significant number of other tools and may not increase the evidential significance (Figure 6.5). If the mark showed a less common size and shape, then this may increase the evidential value to the next level. If we now consider a very unusual type and size of tool on class features only, this may be of more evidential significance than a common type and size of tool. Such a comparison is illustrated in Figure 6.6, where the mark has been made by an implement with a rounded profile, such as the tyre lever shown. Assuming that there is no fine detail present in the mark, even under microscopic examination, the general shape and size of the tool is

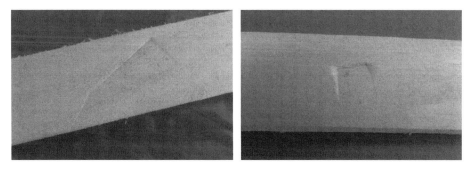

Figure 6.5 Examples of impressed marks, without any fine detail, that have been made by a screwdriver as indicated by the tapering blade (left) and distinct tip (right). This could reduce the number of other tools that could have been responsible to scewdrivers with this shape and size.

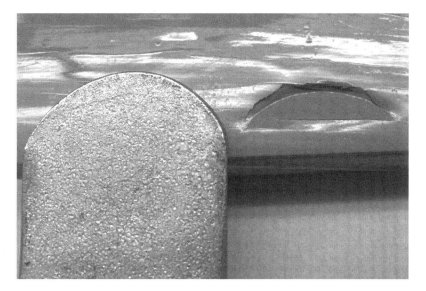

Figure 6.6 A tyre lever with a rounded tip profile (left), shown against a mark of similar profile in painted wood (right) with no fine detail. Other tools that could have been responsible would have to be rounded, which rules out a lot of differently shaped levering tools, offering a moderate level of support.

all there is. All other types of levering tool can be eliminated from having been responsible, and this could strengthen the level of support to a more moderate level. With an even less common tool, such as the 'jaws of life', a hydraulic cutting tool normally used by emergency services personnel to cut apart damaged cars that have been involved in road traffic accidents in order to free a victim, it may be possible to push the evidential significance of the findings to a strong level.

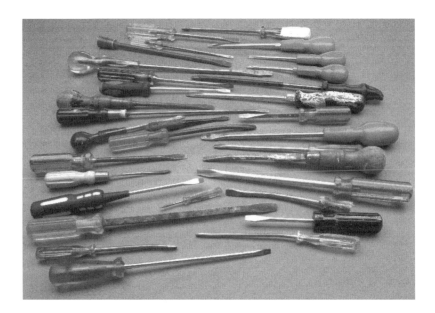

Figure 6.7   A collection of screwdrivers of different sizes and finishes.

Sometimes a comparison will be restricted up to and including sub-class features. For the purposes of interpretation, this sort of feature could include manufactured detail that may be repeated on other tools produced in a similar way (such as specific shape or type of detail, e.g. pressed lines) or those that are not discriminatory enough to be a distinctive feature, for example regular or poorly defined grinding detail. It will not be possible to determine this from purely sliding marks, but some sliding marks contain a small area of partial impression that may contain such detail. A major pitfall in interpretation could be if a sub-class feature is incorrectly assumed to be unique and the type of feature needs to be confirmed before continuing. It is good to know what variations can be expected within different groups of tool type to help evaluate the level of evidence, as some show much less variation in sub-class features. Figure 6.7 shows a collection of screwdrivers of different sizes and finishes. Where a mark also shows the type and size of tool responsible, this again reduces the group of other tools that may have been responsible. This could strengthen the level of support to a *moderate* level. This means that there are fewer tools that could have made the mark than for a limited conclusion, but more than for a strong conclusion. There still remain a middling number of tools that would not correspond to the mark to the same extent as the suspect tool and so the results are still more likely given the prosecution view.

At this point, the following scale of support has been demonstrated as:

1. no support

2. limited support

3. moderate support

4. strong support

5. this tool made the mark (or very strong support).

The scale described has the advantage of flexibility, but does have some problems. One problem is that it implies there are sharp boundaries between the various levels. In practice this is not important, as the required end is to present a reliable indication of the weight of the evidence to the court, which they can relate to all of the other evidence they will hear, in order to reach a final guilty or not guilty verdict. Having a scale, such as the one above, allows the practitioner to have a credible way to do this.

Another problem is that, as we suggested earlier in the chapter and as you can gather from the above discussion, tool marks is an inherently, subjective and opinion-based arena. There is a lack of readily available, reliable data on the commonality of tools and their features with which to inform the evaluation process. What we mean by subjectivity can also be termed 'heuristics' (Champod *et al.*, 2003); this is where an expert uses their experience and knowledge to make a personal judgement about the problem at hand. It could also be known as 'an educated guess'. However, given a similarly broad scale to work with, similarly trained and experienced individuals could be expected to reach a similar level of conclusion. On occasion, there will be differences that may be due to factors such as the ability to visualise the detail being limited by the casting materials and equipment used and differences in experience and knowledge. This also highlights the importance of having a verification process, to ensure that the conclusion given is at the right level, as will be described later in this chapter.

We feel that the scale we have proposed gives a suitable range of conclusions with which to reflect the weight of the evidence. There are other scales in existence for use across a range of forensic disciplines and in different countries, which have more or less gradations, similarly worded or with slight differences. For example, by comparison, The Association of Firearm and

Tool Mark Examiners' (AFTE) range of conclusions includes identification, inconclusive, elimination and unsuitable for comparison (AFTE, 1990). However, for our purposes, this is a fairly limited range. Other scales, where there are more levels similar to those here, such as 'moderately strong', tend to lose meaning and emphasis. Some scales used will have different wording, which describe whether or not the expert thinks the known tool could have made the mark. Scales such as these tend to include the wording 'could, probably, very probably, almost certainly, likely not' for example; however, again, these conclusions do not give an idea of how many other tools could also potentially have left the mark. In 2005, the European Network of Forensic Science Institutes' (ENFSI) Working Group for Marks produced a report that attempted to correlate differently worded scales used by practitioners across Europe, by equating them into six different levels.

6.3   Other considerations

The foregoing has dealt with reasonably well defined marks, albeit some having only limited amounts of detail present, and it is easy to show the correspondence between the crime and control items where the comparison progresses logically from class to sub-class to unique detail. However, in reality this is a fairly simplistic view and there are other considerations that must be taken into account.

It is important not to stop a comparison too early just because a 'link' has been found, albeit at a less than conclusive level. Making and comparing further test marks or comparing a different area of mark and tool may give a better correspondence. To illustrate the change in detail that can be produced as different parts of a tool tip come into contact with a surface, Figure 6.8 shows a striated crime mark compared with different areas along the length of a test mark made with the tool tip at varying angles from the substrate. Figure 6.9 shows two areas of comparison of an impressed mark. In the first comparison, there is a limited area of not very well defined fine parallel lines, which show some level of agreement (and also some differences) to grinding on the surface of the tool. By moving the area of comparison, as the second comparison shows, a better correspondence can be found. In addition to the limited amount of grinding detail (the lines running horizontally), there is also detail corresponding to scratch damage that runs diagonally across the tool surface at differing angles present in the mark. This is more characteristic than the very limited amount of grinding detail alone.

Another consideration is when there are apparent differences between a crime mark and a known item and the examiner has to assess these to determine if they are significant or not. Some differences can be explained simply because unknown and known items are not linked. However, other differences can sometimes be reasonably explained. In these cases, you would

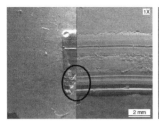
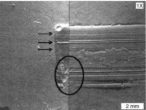
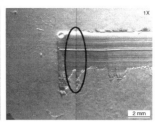

Figure 6.8 Series of comparisons between casts of a scene mark (left half of each photograph) and a test pull mark made using the suspect tool tip (right half of each photograph), which varies in its angle to the substrate as the mark is made. The first photograph shows marks of a similar width, with a small area of matching characteristic detail shown at the bottom; the second photograph shows more detail beginning to match but there is still non-matching detail; the third photograph shows excellent correspondence of most of the striations in the top half of the mark. The change in detail occurs as different features on the tool's tip come into contact with the substrate.

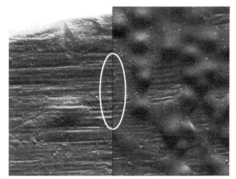
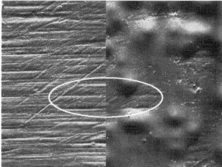

Figure 6.9 Each photograph shows a replica cast of the suspect tool (left half of each photograph) compared with a recast of the scene mark (right half of each photograph). There is heavy interference from the background in the scene mark. The first photograph shows a limited amount of impressed but poorly defined grinding detail that corresponds to the tool, although there is some detail surrounding that indicated which appears different. The second photograph shows a corresponding grinding detail with the addition of scratches running diagonally across the grinding, which is more evidentially significant.

also need a significant amount of other detail to correspond. Take for example, a very rusty chisel with a characteristically damaged tip profile. The mark in question shows a combination of impressed and dynamic detail, the dynamic detail coming from the tip and also the bevelled edge. Comparison shows that the mark was made by a tool of the same size and shape with the same tip profile. The dynamic detail produced by the bevelled edge shows coarse striations that correspond to damage on the surface of the suspect chisel, but there is much more variation in the fine striations in between. On reflection, as the submitted chisel is very rusty, its surface friable (fragile and flaky) and changeable, this observation can be easily explained due to this corrosion and would not necessarily change an expert's opinion of the two showing a significant correspondence in other respects.

Some differences in detail may be because further damage to the tool has occurred after the crime mark was made. The circumstances may allow for that to have happened, for example there is a significant time lapse between the offence and recovery of the tool, there is lots of fresh damage on the tool, or the tool may have been ground after making a mark. In these cases, it could be possible that the suspect tool is responsible, but is now in a substantially different condition than when the mark was made; in this instance a qualified conclusion of 'the mark was not made by the tool in its current condition' may be more appropriate. Sometimes marks may be so limited or variable in their detail due to angle or other such factor that they cannot be reproduced in test marks, meaning it is not possible to rule out the tool in question, but it is not possible to provide any specific link of association either.

Technical difficulties in casting can also limit a comparison or make it more difficult, for example, large bubbles being trapped during casting. Where detail is unobscured and therefore does not affect the comparison or level of conclusion, such as in Figure 6.1, this is not an issue. However, sometimes fairly large areas can be missing as illustrated in Figure 6.10 and may lead to a downgrading of the evidence.

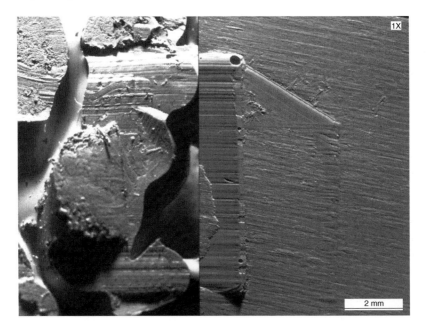

Figure 6.10 Cast of a scene mark that has large voids (left), severely limiting the amount of detail visible for comparison with a cast of a test mark made using the suspect tool tip (right). However, in this instance, the limited detail at the outer edges of the scene mark that can be compared corresponds to the test mark.

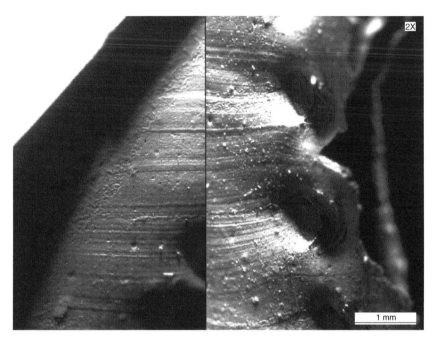

Figure 6.11 Comparison of casts of a test mark in a tyre (left) with a stab mark from a damaged tyre (right). There is excellent correspondence of detail, particularly the coarser striations, given the stretchy nature of the tyre rubber and action used has created some curvature and distortion.

How the mark has been made and in what type of surface must also be considered. For example, Figure 6.11 shows a stab mark. If attention is only focused on the features present, one can see that there are striations in common, but also some apparent differences, which could superficially suggest that the result will be less than conclusive. What has not been taken into account is the material that the mark is made in; the mark has been made in tyre rubber. This introduces a number of different matters for consideration. The flexible consistency of the rubber allows the tool to expand the rubber as it enters, with a resulting contraction when it is removed. This will be difficult to reproduce and the examiner should not expect an exact alignment of the striae formed. Next, rubbery materials do not easily form fine striations and usually only the coarser striations are reliable. Lastly, a stabbing action is not normally totally vertical to the object and there is some curvature both in the action and the mark. By taking these factors into account, and by making some small adjustments in the x, y and z planes of the comparator, which can also include rotations to show that there is good agreement in the relative, if not the absolute, arrangement of the striations, it becomes apparent that there is a very high level of agreement, leading to the conclusion that the submitted knife made the mark.

6.4   Verification

So far in this book we have dealt with the first three elements of the ACE-V process mentioned in Chapter 1. The Analysis, Comparison and Evaluation have all been carried out. This can all be done by one person, the court reporting scientist (with the help of assistant examiners if necessary), who will give testimony in court if later required. This individual will be 'The Prosecution Expert' and that person has to be confident that they can justify their evidence. However, in most cases that person will not, and should not, have completed the case in isolation. Whenever possible the fourth element of ACE-V should be undertaken before any case is reported. As given in Chapter 1, Verification (often also known as a 'critical findings check') is an independent examination, by another qualified practitioner, which critically reviews the findings.

If there are three or more court reporting scientists in the laboratory it should be possible to carry out the verification procedure. At the end of the examination, the reporting scientist records their findings, including the evaluation, and has their work reviewed by one of their colleagues. This colleague should not only be a qualified court reporting scientist in their own right, but should also have been trained and assessed as a person qualified to carry out a critical findings check. The requirements of the verification process were given in Chapter 1, but bear reiteration here. The process should ensure that:

• The examiner has followed the appropriate documented examination process and applied the appropriate and relevant scientific methodology and techniques.

• The work and findings of the examination are reflected in the conclusion reported. The results must support the conclusion and clearly there should be no understatement or overstatement of the findings.

• The maximum evidence has been obtained, that nothing has been overlooked and there are no other marks that may change the outcome.

• The submitting authority's question has been fully addressed.

This will involve more than just looking at the match found by the examiner. The verifier should look at the paperwork with the submission, the tool, the original mark and the range of test marks made and other materials used, where that is appropriate. They may even wish to make their own test mark. It should be stressed that it not being suggested that the full examination is repeated but the verifier should be in a position to provide an independent confirmation of the evaluation. What is happening is basically the same as a peer review of a paper for a scientific journal. When this has been done, the verifier should, as a minimum, sign and date the notes to say that they agree with the evaluation. Preferably, they will separately document their findings and evaluation prior to reading the documentation and conclusion reached by the reporting scientist. If there is a disagreement then another qualified person acts as an arbitrator.

Although a verification process could, theoretically be carried out in house where there are only two court reporting scientists, this should be discouraged as they would be checking each other's work all the time and this could lead to problems, with no third party to check that they are consistently examining and reporting to a correct standard. When there is only one qualified court reporting scientist, consideration should be given to making suitable arrangements with other organisations to get the work and findings checked independently.

In addition to having the examination, findings and evaluation checked, all reports and judicial statements should be checked before leaving the laboratory to ensure that:

- They deal with all the questions asked by the submitting authority.

- A proper record has been made of the examination needed to answer those questions.

- The report/statement is fully supported by the findings of the examination.

- All relevant information surrounding the examination, interpretation and evaluation (including information used and any assumptions that have been made) are disclosed.

The statement/report should include an evaluation of the recorded results. Where detailing the evaluation makes the report/statement too long, it can be added as an appendix to the main document and could include images of the match(es) found.

6.5 After the examination

When the examination and verification process is complete there is still a need to maintain continuity of materials. The examiner should repackage and return all the submitted materials. They should also securely package and either return or retain any relevant materials such as casts, test marks or contact traces that were made or removed during the examination. There should be full documentation as to what has happened to the items and materials.

6.6   Quality assurance

The basic requirements for quality assurance were given in Chapter 1. These primarily relate to the situation applying in England and Wales at the time of writing. These may change with future legislation or codes of practice and practitioners working in other jurisdictions will have to consider the requirements in their own countries.

Nevertheless, it is clear from the above that there is a subjective element in the interpretation and evaluation of the findings from tool mark comparisons. These subjective elements need to be controlled, in as far as it is possible to do so. It is not a unique problem confined to tool mark examination and similar practices have developed in other scientific disciplines where recognising characteristic morphological features is important (Boyer *et al.*, 2011).

As already mentioned, one step towards controlling the subjectivity is to have a written set of procedures for undertaking an examination. The intent is to produce a document, or set of documents that allows a dependable examination and evaluation of the materials submitted to be carried out. The procedures are not intended to act like a factory production line where items are feed in at one end and an evaluation appears at the other. Nor are they intended to rigidly constrain the examination; where there is a need to vary the procedure this should be possible, but the changes must be recorded and recognised in the subsequent evaluation. The changed procedure must also be shown to be capable of giving equivalent results to the normal procedures. Very often the procedures will have been assessed by a recognised outside body as being fit for the examination undertaken. While the procedures undertaken by different organisations can vary, they should ideally reflect best practice in the relevant field, allowing for the circumstances under which the examinations will be carried out (e.g. as given under Section 6.4, Verification, different arrangements may be required for organisations with only one or two qualified examiners). More importantly, these documents should be reviewed periodically to ensure that they are up-to-date and reflect any changes to procedures that can improve the examination and evaluation.

Another way to demonstrate that work is being delivered consistently and to a required standard is to participate in declared and undeclared trials organised by recognised institutions. Such institutions include the European Network of Forensic Science Institutes' (ENFSI) Working Group for Marks. A declared trial is one where materials are given to the participant, who is normally asked to examine them and evaluate the findings as they would in a normal case, but they are fully aware that this is a trial. An undeclared trial is one where the materials are submitted as normal for a case of that type, such that the scientist is unaware that it is a trial, but the organisers know what outcome to expect from the examination. In general what these trials have shown is that, provided the examiners are using the same scale for evaluation, scientists working in different organisations come to similar levels of conclusions (with any differences due to factors as described earlier). That is, given the correct training and despite the subjectivity, different individuals are able to reach evaluative conclusions that are consistent with the expectations of the organisers setting the trials.

References

AFTE (1990).Theory of identification, range of striae comparison reports and modified glossary definitions – An AFTE criteria for identification committee report. *AFTE Journal*, **22** (3), 275–279.

Aitken, C.G.G. (1995) *Statistics and the Evaluation of Evidence for Forensic Scientists (Statistics in Practice)*, John Wiley & Sons, Ltd, Chichester.

Biedermann, A., Taroni, F. and Champod, C. (2012) How to assign a likelihood ratio in a footwear mark case: An analysis and discussion in the light of R v T. law, probability and risk. *Law, Probability and Risk*, **11**, 259–277

Boyer, D.M., Lipman, Y., St Clair, E., *et al.* (2011) Algorithms to automatically quantify the geometric similarity of anatomical surfaces. *Proceedings of the National Academy of Sciences of the United States of America*, **108** (45), 18221–18226.

Champod, C., Baldwin, D., Taroni, F. and Buckleton, J.S (2003) Firearm and tool marks' identification: The Bayesian approach. . *Association of Firearm and Tool Mark Examiners' (AFTE) Journal*, **35**, 307–316.

ENFSI (2005) *Conclusion Scale for Interpreting Findings in Proficiency Tests and Collaborative Exercises within the WG Marks*, http://www.poliisi.fi/intermin/hankkeet/wgm/home.nsf/files/Harmonized_Conclusion_Scale_of_EWGM/$file/Harmonized_Conclusion_Scale_of_EWGM.pdf (accessed October 2012).

Association of Forensic Science Providers (2009) Standards for the formulation of evaluative forensic science expert opinion. *Science and Justice*, **49** (3), 161–164.

Stoney, D.A. (1991) What made us ever think we could individualize using statistics? *Journal of the Forensic Science Society*, **31** (2), 197–199.

7
Manufacturing Marks: Involving Tool Mark Related Examinations

7.1 Introduction

Manufacturing 'marks' can be found on a whole range of mass produced and widely distributed items, resulting from either detail on the machine tools and other equipment used to form and finish the product, or the materials used to make the product. In general, they are considered to be minor flaws in the finished articles, although the features do not normally result in the item failing quality control, as they do not adversely affect either the performance or the overall appearance of the product. In a forensic context, these manufactured flaws, which are often microscopic, provide a powerful means to discriminate between different sources and batches of manufactured products.

In this chapter, we will focus on four examples of items that we feel illustrate the main points of this type of examination, which can be applied to other similar items, and the type of marks that are likely to be encountered. The items that we will discuss are screws, insulated cable, copied coins and security ties. These items may be recovered in a wide variety of criminal cases. For example, screws and insulated cable could be from a terrorist case, copied coins in cases involving allegations of fraud and security ties from customs' and excise cases to secure a variety of containers with illicit contents.

Usually the case requirement is to see if there is any evidence to link something in the suspect's possession or at their premises to a scene or to see if scenes are linked. Therefore, it is best for the crime scene examiner to collect all possible samples at the time they investigate the scene(s). It is much easier to review the items after they have been taken away from the location where

The Forensic Examination and Interpretation of Tool Marks, First Edition.
David Baldwin, John Birkett, Owen Facey and Gilleon Rabey.
© 2013 John Wiley & Sons, Ltd. Published 2013 by John Wiley & Sons, Ltd.

they have been found and it may not be known at the time what relevance the items have until the laboratory examination begins. Items such as screws and cable ties may still be contained in retail packets and it is important to consider the recovery of opened and unused retail packs. It may be necessary to purchase other retail packs to obtain information about distribution.

The basic principles that underpin tool mark comparison are also directly applicable to the effective comparison of manufacturing marks, as the comparison requires an understanding of background information on exactly how such marks are produced, and how they are likely to vary among items produced by the same overall process. The examination of manufacturing marks involves the interpretation of the macroscopic features of the article, to determine how it was made, and then to deduce what characteristic detail may be present, visualise it and carry out a meaningful comparison. In many cases a comparison of physical features is often easier to do and can provide at least as strong, if not stronger, evidence than chemical analyses of the composition of the type of materials involved, such as plastic or metal.

As with the examination of tool marks, described in previous chapters, where there is microscopic detail, a bench microscope should be used to undertake an initial examination and assess what detail is present. The casting of this detail to facilitate a more thorough examination and the use of a comparator will also be necessary. The major points of interest here are how to prepare the marks so that they can be compared and what significance can be attached to matching marks.

7.2 Screws

Screws are produced in vast numbers on a production line, where the head is moulded from the end of metal wire, using a forging process to shape the head and introduce the slot where the screwdriver will insert (Figure 7.1). A grip mark can be formed on the shank at this time and there may be impressed marks in the slot and on the face of the screw head. The screw may then be gripped in a clamp, underneath the head on the shank (Figure 7.2), so that the screw threads can be cut. Another method of forming the screw thread is to send them through a rolling device to shape rather than cut them, which means that there is no waste material (swarf), and this is often preferable to the manufacturer. This process work hardens the surface of the thread, meaning that it will 'bite' better into the substrate it is used on. Impressed marks on the head and grip marks underneath, plus any cutting detail on the thread, can be useful features to compare between screws. Owing to the repeating actions involved, they will change over time due to wear and tear of the machine parts involved.

The screws will end up in hoppers and are put into boxes for distribution. The order of manufacture is not preserved after production, so the screws

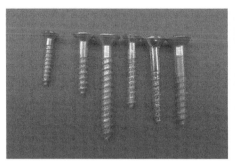
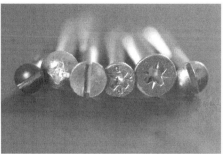

Figure 7.1 A selection of screws (left) and variation in slots on screw heads (right).

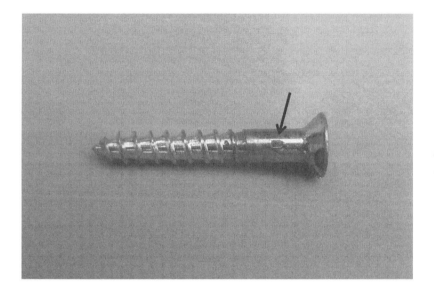

Figure 7.2 Rectangular grip mark, indicated on screw shank.

could come from widely different times from the same production line or from different lines altogether, but still end up in the same retail pack. Questions that may be asked in cases involving screws could be of the ilk 'Is the screw used in explosive device A the same as the one used in device B?' or 'Did the screws from the scene come from this retail pack found at the suspect's home address?' The evaluation can be very complex and will often be limited by the amount of information available about the production methods and distribution of the items.

If we have a scenario where we have two screws, from different locations, the question could be 'Did the two screws come from the same source?' A detailed comparison of the detail on the two screws has been undertaken and the findings show that they bear the same manufacturing detail. In response to the question asked, it may be that all we can say is that the two screws have been produced on the same manufacturing line. In this situation, either the marks produced are simply class features that apply to the bulk of the items made, or there will be differences between every object, but there is no way of showing how the differences vary with time because no other screws are available. There is debate as to whether this is a helpful comment, as it does not really give any assessment of the evidential significance, but this may be all that can be said.

If the scenario changes, you could now have a number of questioned screws and a retail pack, which has been opened and is missing some of its contents. In this instance, the question is 'Did the screws come from the retail pack?' The scientist will be considering whether or not the questioned screws are likely to have come from the distribution of screws in the pack. This will involve a much more complex examination, with the examiner looking at the population of (or a representative sample, depending on how many there are) screws from the questioned sample and retail pack, to see if each population profile corresponds. The examination will entail considerations such as whether all the screws show the same or different detail, or whether there is the same variation in detail on different screws. Here the examiner will have to assess the detail and look at how well the detail matches. Where there is no correspondence of the population profiles, it seems likely that the screws and retail pack are unrelated and another retail pack would show a better correspondence.

A consideration in some cases, where there is a low level of correspondence between the population profiles, is that there is a possibility of the screws being unrelated and the fact that there is some correspondence is a chance occurrence. A more rigorous approach would make use of statistical analysis to determine the level of correspondence between the two or more samples. Nonparametric statistics can be useful here, especially its version of the chi squared test, but describing this falls outside the scope of this book. Standard texts on nonparametric statistics, such as Corder and Foreman (2009) can be consulted for further information.

Similar principles can be applied to the examination and evaluation of items such as nails, bolts and so on, although the detail being looked at could alter depending on the item (Figure 7.3).

7.3   Insulated cable

Molten plastic, as used to insulate cables, is drawn out through an annular die, which can leave striated lines on the solid plastic coating's surface, known as extrusion detail. Metal used to produce wires and cables is also treated in a similar way by being drawn through a die to decrease its diameter. This process can leave striated lines on the surface of the metal. Such detail can

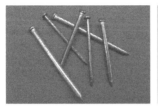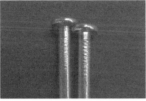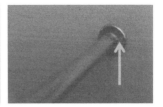

Figure 7.3 A selection of nails (left); grip marks underneath nail heads (middle); flash detail under the head of a nail from a closed die forging process (right).

also be found on plastic and metal tubing and piping and is capable of being cast for comparison.

Questions that are asked in cases involving insulated cable are along the lines of 'Did this length of cable come from this roll or a much larger piece?' The examination could involve a physical fit, where a potential fit could be supported by corresponding manufacturing detail; however, this type of examination is covered in more detail in Chapter 8. Here, we will discuss where no physical fit has been possible, for example there is a missing piece or the ends have been soldered or exploded, and so an assessment needs to be made of how well the manufacturing detail alone corresponds.

In these cases, it is necessary to estimate how the marks change along the length of the items, so that any correspondence between the marks can be properly evaluated. In those cases where there are a number of manufacturers, being able to say that a questioned item was manufactured on the same line as the known item may have some evidential value to the court.

7.4 Copied coins

In cases involving copied coins, it is paramount to verify with the investigating officer exactly what the charge is going to be, and the reporting scientist may also need to liaise with a professional numismatist (a coin collector) to get all the facts before proceeding. This is of more relevance to the charge than the mark examination itself, as cases involving fraud and fake items can be fraught with danger for the innocent forensic scientist to wander into. For example, in cases of collectible coins, it is up to the buyer to verify that items are what the seller says they are, because if they turn out to be copies, then there is no recourse even if the seller knew. Another example is that it is illegal to melt or otherwise tamper with coins bearing the monarch's head (current or past) in the United Kingdom; however, it may not be illegal to tamper with another Commonwealth state's coinage in the United Kingdom.

As interesting as this all is, the most frequently submitted types of copied coins in the United Kingdom are one pound (£1) Sterling coins. Since their introduction by the Royal Mint in the early 1980s, the methods used to produce copied £1 coins has developed and it has become increasingly difficult to determine whether they are genuine or not. Originally, copied coins (not just £1, but 50p coins as well) were very crude, usually being cast to approximately the correct size in white metal (or lead) and then metal removed by drilling or filing to produce a 'token' of the correct weight for use in vending machines. Having been obviously copied, such coins did not usually require examination by a marks' expert. A marks' expert was normally called in when the equipment, usually simple plaster moulds with obvious characteristic detail, had been recovered. The examination was carried out as for most impressed marks, taking casts of the moulds as necessary to compare with the tokens.

Silicone rubber moulds were next to be used, again casting the coins with white metal. If 'gold' coins were being made, these may have been painted gold after casting, although this was not always the case. Initial testing was simple; scratching the gold surface to see what metal had been used. It was then often required that coins from different seizures would be compared against each other to see if there was a common source. Although not so prone to damage after production, the rubber moulds would reproduce the fine damage detail present on the original coin that was used to make the mould. This detail would then potentially be reproduced on all coins produced in that mould.

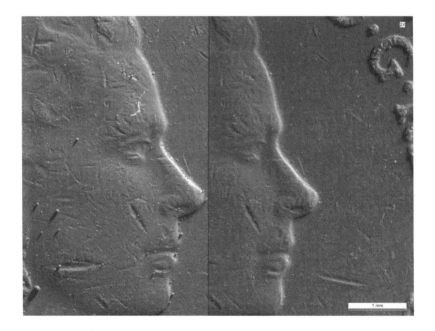

Figure 7.4   Repeated mould detail on two copied one pound Sterling coins.

More recently coins have been struck in the same way as genuine currency. This is to say that a blank is cut from a strip of metal then introduced into a machine where the obverse and reverse designs are stamped onto the surfaces. The stamping process means that any imperfections in the dies will be transferred to the coins produced from them, and this can be compared either between coins from different sources or between the dies and coins. The examination of coins is usually carried out to determine whether or not they are genuine, or to determine if they have been made using certain pieces of equipment. Having established that any damage detail from a mould was not part of the original design (by consulting information provided by the Royal Mint), the scientist could then determine that the coins had a common origin (Figure 7.4), as no two genuine coins would have randomly acquired the same damage.

7.5 Security ties/tags

Security ties are often referred to as cable ties or ratchet ties (Figure 7.5). However, those used specifically for security may have additional features, such as a security number printed or moulded onto the head of the tie. These are produced using multiple machines, in a process called 'injection moulding'. An injection mould may have multiple cavities so that several copies of the article are produced simultaneously at each pass. Each mould

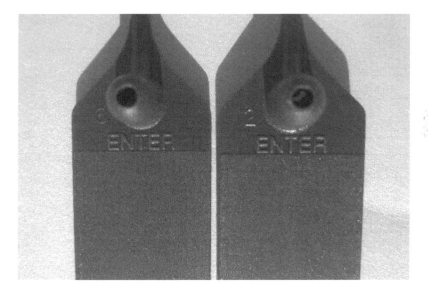

Figure 7.5   The numbers, lettering and fine surface texture of two ratchet tags, relate to the mould cavities in which they were made.

unit may have imperfections from damage, or may have been ground, or have an engraved number associated with it. This means that items produced from the same unit will have the same mould detail on their surface. In some moulding processes, inserts may be introduced into the mould to change some aspect, such a logo. The insert may have different locations within the mould for different batches.

Molten plastic is injected into the mould through 'gates' near the head end. Detail relating specifically to the moulding process may occur, such as the introduction of air bubbles or 'flow' lines where the molten material has flowed and set. These could occur at random or with particular designs they may occur in similar positions between pieces. The head end of a security tie may also show injection detail, where the molten material was injected into the mould through the gate.

All may potentially provide useful discriminating information, although the head usually has the best detail on it. Questions asked are usually along similar lines as for screws concerning a common source or having come from a particular retail pack. Evaluations involving distributions and population profiles could be necessary. A retail packet of cable ties could show a variety of ties from different moulds. For example, the cable ties could be numbered 1, 2, 3, 4 and 5. The questioned cable ties could be 8, 9, which could suggest they were from another source, or they could be numbers 2 and 5, which could provide a moderate level of corroborative evidence. It would be good in these cases to look at other packets of cable ties from the manufacturer/distributor to see the variation and give some background information to the expert with which to make a more informed judgement. The evaluation proceeds along similar lines to that used for screws and similar items.

Reference

Corder, G.W. and Foreman, D.I. (2009) *Nonparametric Statistics for Non-Statisticians: A Step-by-Step Approach*, John Wiley & Sons, Inc., Hoboken.

8
Physical Fits: Involving Tool Mark Related Examinations

8.1 Introduction

'Physical fits', often referred to as 'mechanical fits', can be encountered in a wide range of forensic examinations, including as part of a more general tool mark case. A physical fit examination is required when it is necessary to show that two, or more, pieces of material, which have been broken, torn, cut or otherwise separated, were originally joined or fitted together. The alternative scenarios being that:

- The pieces are obviously different from each other and therefore unrelated.

- They appear similar but do not fit back together, in which case this may indicate that they are from the same item but for some reasonable explanation do not fit and additional features may have to be used to form a conclusion.

- They do not fit back together because they are pieces of similar but unrelated items.

Various features of the items may be used for the comparison, depending on the category the fit falls into. These categories will be described below.

The Forensic Examination and Interpretation of Tool Marks, First Edition.
David Baldwin, John Birkett, Owen Facey and Gilleon Rabey.
© 2013 John Wiley & Sons, Ltd. Published 2013 by John Wiley & Sons, Ltd.

The word 'broken' is used here to imply that the material is thick enough to 'snap' or 'crack' and will leave an irregular edge with fracture detail on it. Typical materials for examination that can have broken edges include knife blades, levering tools, sheet glass, bottles or vehicle wing mirrors and other fittings. Occasionally, irregularly cut surfaces, such as from a sawn shotgun barrel or sawn bones from a dismembered body, can be examined using the same techniques as used for broken surfaces, as will be described later in this chapter. In contrast, 'torn' implies a thin material where only an irregular edge can be seen. Such materials could include plastic film, fabric or paper; those relating more to marks' examinations, for example plastic film, will be described in more detail in Chapter 9.

The skills, knowledge and forensic expertise required to undertake a physical fit examination will vary depending on the material being examined and the complexity of the examination. An example is the examination of torn clothing where the expertise required relates to fibres and fabrics and so would not typically be carried out by a marks' examiner.

It would be impossible to cover all possibilities in this book, so in this chapter we will explain the general categories of physical fits and provide some examples. As with the rest of the book, this will focus on physical fits that are more closely related to marks' examination. For simplicity, we will assume that the submitted items have been initially examined and determined to be suitable for comparison, that is, there are no obvious differences.

As stated in the Introduction of the book, physical fit examinations can, for convenience, be separated into the following categories.

1. Broken items that can obviously be fitted back together; otherwise known as 'jigsaw' fits. A tool mark examiner would not necessarily be required to demonstrate this sort of physical fit.

2. Broken items where the pieces require routine tool mark examination techniques to demonstrate if the pieces fit together or otherwise correspond, and thus to form a conclusion. The detail may require use of casting and a microscopic comparison.

3. Broken, torn or cut items, where knowledge of manufacture and type of marks left on the surface of the item need to be taken into account in order to support a fit. Typically, these sorts of examinations require techniques more commonly associated with routine tool mark examinations or manufacturing marks, particularly those relating to plastic film items.

4. Items that were originally fitted together or were in contact for a period of time. Typically, these examinations involve a consideration of what material has been transferred or the effect of the contact.

There will be situations where the lines between the first three categories are blurred, so they can only be considered as a guide.

8.2 Scene examination

There are a wide variety of circumstances where parts of broken and cut items, or those that have been in contact for a period of time, may be left at a scene. Examples of such items could include:

- Tool tips that have broken off may be found on the ground, possibly mixed in with other debris lying around at the scene or lodged in a forced door or window.

- Cut insulated cables or wires.

- Other parts of tools that could have broken off, such as a knife handle becoming detached from its blade and tang.

- Objects or broken keys that have become lodged in a keyway.

- Miscellaneous items consisting of two or more pieces that may have been used as a weapon, such as a ceramic ornament, bottle or piece of wood. A physical fit comparison in this instance would be to determine what the full item looked like or to fit it back to other pieces that may have been found elsewhere.

- Pieces of masonry, bricks and so on, for example that have been used to weigh down a body in water, for comparison against a wall or similar, using features such as the shape of broken mortar.

- Flakes of paint that have chipped off an item.

The corresponding parts of the original item may be found at different locations and so require a physical fit examination to link them. For example, a knife may be in the suspect's possession, while the tip is found embedded in the victim. It may also happen that pieces recovered from a scene need to be fitted together to reconstruct the original item that has been used in an attack on a victim.

Sometimes, a potential physical fit examination is identified whilst examining items submitted in cases involving different disciplines, for example clothing being examined for paint or glass could reveal a fragment large enough to be fitted back to the 'control'.

A point to be kept in mind is that it is not the sizes of fractured surfaces that are important, but the quality of the detail present. Good results can be obtained from areas that are less than 1 mm square. Therefore, it is not advisable to try and remove embedded items from their surrounds at the scene, but to cut or otherwise remove the item together with part of the surround. Where broken items, such as bottles, are concerned it is important to collect all the material present. Packaging the pieces to minimise any further breaking is also important.

8.3   Categories of physical fit and laboratory examination

8.3.1   Jigsaw fits

These are broken items that can be obviously fitted back together; hence the name 'jigsaw' fits. These are normally large pieces that, as the name suggests, fit together like a jigsaw, to give a two- or three-dimensional item and may consist of many pieces. The pieces have an irregular shape with edges that have a visible characteristic profile, which enables pieces to be readily put back together (Figure 8.1). Often the surface will also have detail on it, such as a pattern, name or texture, which also helps show the matching location of the pieces.

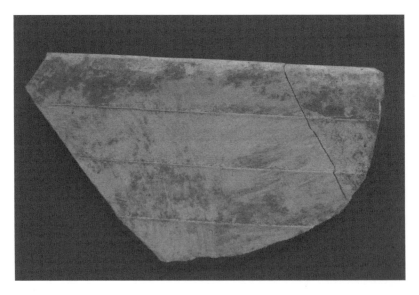

Figure 8.1   A physical fit of two pieces of broken pot, note the 'jigsaw' fit of the broken edges, with parallel lines on each piece matching up.

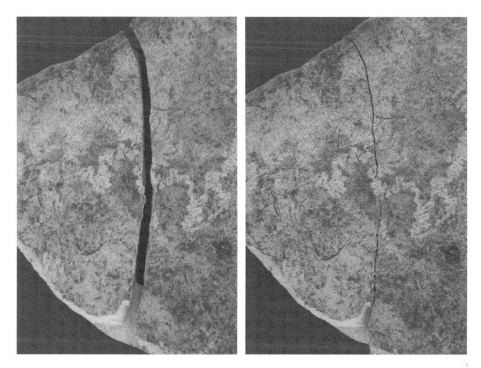

Figure 8.2   The reverse of the physical fit shown in Figure 8.1, note the patterning of dirt and mould that crosses over the join.

This category of fit is normally associated with materials such as metal, china, hard plastic and wood. The laboratory requirements for this type of physical fit examination are to have good lighting and a sufficiently large workspace. The examiner should clearly and permanently mark, as far as possible, the known and questioned items so that they can be distinguished before starting the examination. Note any features that could aid in finding the matching broken surface, for example curvature, lines or marks crossing breaks (Figure 8.2). The pieces and potential fits should be photographically recorded and there should be a consistent system used for joining the pieces together.

8.3.1.1   Multiple broken pieces   In situations where there are multiple pieces of a broken object for a jigsaw type fit, it will be necessary to fit them all back together to provide the evidence. Such evidence may be sent for laboratory examination because the investigating officer does not have the resources available to undertake fitting the pieces together, or because an official forensic examination is preferred to demonstrate the fit.

Fractures involved in this sort of physical fit examination are broadly of the more 'brittle' type. These occur in materials such as ceramic and glass, where small pieces of material splinter from the surface of the propagating fracture so that the two surfaces formed no longer exactly correspond. There may also be generic similarities between the surfaces formed in a brittle fracture that depend on the speed of the crack propagation. This can present some problems, but generally can be worked around where pieces are large enough.

In the situation where there are only one or two broken edges to be fitted back together, then a detailed examination of the broken surfaces may be required, depending on how characteristic the profile of the broken edge(s) were or if they were distorted. An initial point for consideration is whether the broken surface was formed by a ductile or brittle fracture. Ductile fractures normally occur in materials such as metals and, while there may have been some distortion, the two surfaces formed mirror images. Brittle fractures occur in materials such as glass and present two different problems. Firstly, small pieces of material may splinter off from the surface of the propagating fracture so that the two surfaces formed no longer exactly correspond. Secondly, there are generic similarities between the surfaces formed in brittle fracture that depend on the speed of the crack propagation. A larger area of fracture surface is therefore needed for this type of comparison compared with that for a ductile fracture surface.

There is usually no quick way to find all the fits; it is useful to discuss with the investigating officer how many of the pieces need to be fitted together if the process is very slow. The reconstructed item needs to be as solid as possible and carefully photographed before packaging in a secure way. No matter how well the item is preserved and packed in its reconstructed form, there is always the possibility that before reaching the court it will have suffered some mishap and become broken. At least the photographs will be available if, on removing the packaging in the witness box, all that is found is a broken mess.

8.3.2   Physical fits requiring tool mark skills

These are broken items where the pieces require routine tool mark examination techniques and principles to be applied in order to demonstrate if the pieces fit together or otherwise correspond and to form a conclusion.

This particular type of physical fit has the essential requirement that the object is made of a material that allows it to break, leaving an irregular, fractured edge as with jigsaw fits. In these particular types of physical fits though, the edge profile may appear uncharacteristic to the naked eye, unlike jigsaw fits, or has been distorted during fracture so the edge profile cannot be compared easily; the fracture detail is often microscopic.

Commonly encountered physical fits that fall into this category include broken tool blades and shafts, where the tool has been unable to withstand the forces being applied and will break, usually due to a defect or weakness

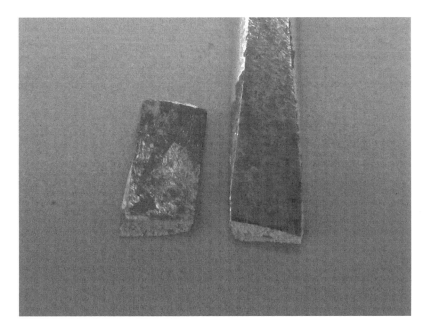

Figure 8.3 A screwdriver with a broken tip.

in the metal (Figure 8.3). Whilst in some cases it may be possible to carry out a jigsaw fit, this generally does not happen in practice, as the broken edge profile may appear fairly uniform and uncharacteristic to the naked eye, even though when viewed microscopically it is often characteristic. Further, more detailed examination will be necessary in order to be satisfied of any conclusive link and to demonstrate it.

Ductile fractures normally occur in materials such as metals and, while there may have been some distortion, the two surfaces formed mirror images. For example, pronounced features on one surface will fit into corresponding hollows on the other and vice versa. A smaller area of fracture surface is therefore usually needed for this type of comparison than that required for brittle fractures.

The best way of comparing the fracture detail is to cast one of the broken surfaces and to make a replica cast of the other. Since the two fracture surfaces of a break will show a mirror image (negative or reverse) of the detail upon them, where they were once joined, it is necessary to get all of the features in the same orientation in order to compare like with like, as shown in Figure 8.4. Owing to the nature of the detail it is always best to use a comparator to do a full comparison. This approach can be applied to all sizes of fracture surfaces provided it is possible to cast them. Sometimes the nature of the surface will require painting on the casting compound or use of a vacuum desiccator to replicate very fine detail without air bubbles.

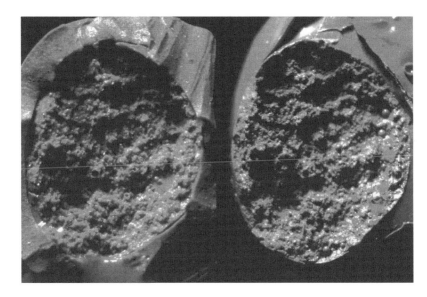

Figure 8.4   A comparison of like with like representations of the fracture surfaces of a broken metal rod.

The two surfaces of the cast and replica may be directly compared using a comparator; the exact method used will depend on the model available. It is also possible to use a macro photographic system or scanning electron microscopy, as previously described in Chapter 5, to carry out a comparison, should it be required.

8.3.3   Physical fits requiring knowledge of manufacturing detail

These are broken, torn or cut items where knowledge of their manufacture and the type of marks that will be left on the surface of the item need to be taken into account in order to support a fit. As we have mentioned already, torn plastic film items will be covered in Chapter 9.

This type of physical fit is frequently encountered. The detail that is present will of course depend on the material under examination, but there is a requirement that, whatever may be present, the scientist understands what the detail is so that they can assess the significance of whether it matches or not from piece to piece. Whether the detail is random damage or manufacturing detail will potentially affect its evidential significance and therefore the outcome of the comparison, but with either type it can be invaluable.

8.3.3.1   Broken items   For broken items where the fractured surfaces have become distorted, the comparison can be difficult, especially if the edge

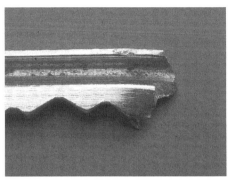 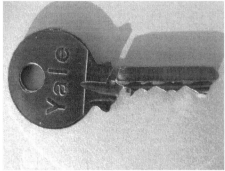

Figure 8.5   The distorted end of a broken key blade (left) and compared with a broken bow (right).

profile is not characteristic. In these situations it is often possible to obtain a potential physical fit between the pieces of material, but there is insufficient clear detail to be able to say definitely that the pieces were once joined. In these situations it may be possible to confirm the fit if the surface detail corresponds across the break. For example, where an incorrect key is used to try to force a lock, the key may break off in the lock. On many occasions this can result in the broken ends having characteristic fracture detail, but this is almost invariably distorted and may need to be supported by additional corresponding features, such as fracture surface detail (Figure 8.5).

8.3.3.2 Cut items   It is possible to separate cut edges into two general categories. First we will consider those instances where there has been no material lost along the cut edge; for example, insulated cables or wires that have been cut into pieces using a sharp cutting tool or blade.

The cut may be at an angle and in some cases the cut ends will show characteristic damage features along the free end. However, this is not always the case and in some instances the cut is straight across the width of the wire so that other pieces of wire with similar straight cut edges cannot be easily distinguished on first inspection. Nevertheless, in many of these situations it is possible to use such features as width, colour, surface texture of the plastic, extrusion detail and striations lines on the surface (as discussed in Chapter 7) together with any detail produced by the cutting tool, to show that pieces of cut wire were originally one continuous length (Figure 8.6). Casting techniques can be used on extrusion, striated and cut detail, then compared using a comparator.

Another situation relates to those occasions where a saw is used to cut the item. By its nature, the use of a saw on wood or metal removes a section of material but it is still possible to show that pieces of gun barrel were originally from a shotgun or that a catalytic converter has been cut from a

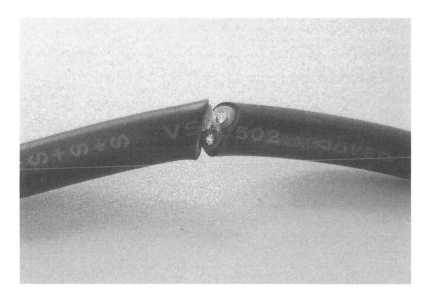

Figure 8.6   Pieces of cut insulated cable.

car. In these situations there is a need to not only consider the general profile of the cut ends and the cut detail that is present, but also to use any surface detail, which may consist of manufacturing detail such as mould features, damage, surface blemishes, labelling and so on. An example of a sawn bolt is shown in Figure 8.7. These can be of considerable assistance to confirming orientation and assisting in assessing whether there is sufficient detail to enable a conclusive association to be established.

8.3.4   Contact 'fits'

This is an examination that can show that two items have been fitted together or that an item has been in one particular location for a period of time. Clearly, by their definition this is not a true a situation where an item has been broken, torn or cut into pieces, but is an examination of other features to support that they have been in contact, such as material that has transferred from one to the other or a characteristic outline has been left.

   This type of examination is well demonstrated by showing that a knife handle and a knife blade that have been found in different locations were originally part of the same knife. Depending on how the handle was attached may determine the type of detail present, but this could include location of rivet holes, any characteristic profile left where the hilt was (which could be dirty or have food in it for example) or by glue used to stick the tang in place. There may even be 'impressed' detail from the knife blade left in glue that

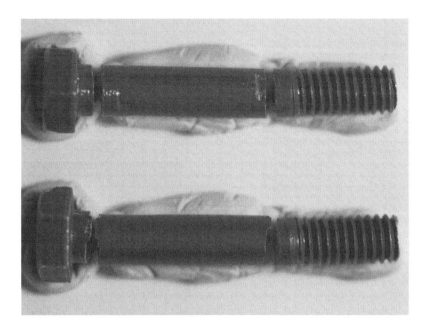

Figure 8.7   Sawn pieces of bolt. Initial cuts (top) and final cuts (bottom).

has set around it inside the handle, such as sheared detail where the blade was blanked out.

This type of examination could also be used to show that a wheel was originally fitted to a specific vehicle's hub. In this particular examination, it is the consideration of factors such as the rust and paint points of contact. Very often there is irregular characteristic detail present, such as the profile of the rust or potential transfer of paint fragments, but all can be used to show that a particular wheel fitted to a hub. Another example is where missing bricks or stones from a wall could be fitted back using mortar locations (Figure 8.8).

Fragmented paint from the surface of a painted tool is one type of fit that potentially spans several of these categories of physical fit. If a fragment is large enough, it can have an obvious shape that can be fitted back like a jigsaw piece to the submitted tool (Figure 8.9). However, this may need to be supported by detail on the back of the fragment, such as grinding or other manufactured detail on the tool (Figure 8.10). This evidence of contact can be demonstrated by using tool mark examination techniques.

8.4   Evaluation

It is very difficult to provide hard and fast rules as to how much detail needs to be present before concluding that the pieces originally formed a single item or

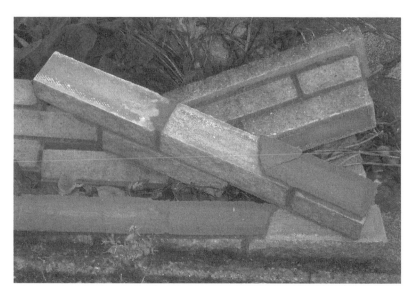

Figure 8.8   A broken wall showing mortar that could be used to carry out a physical fit examination.

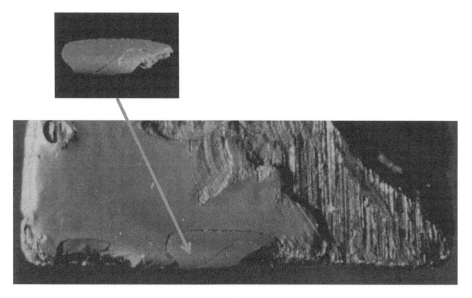

Figure 8.9   The main picture shows a physical fit of a fragment of paint recovered from the scene (top left) to an area of missing paint on the surface of the submitted tool.

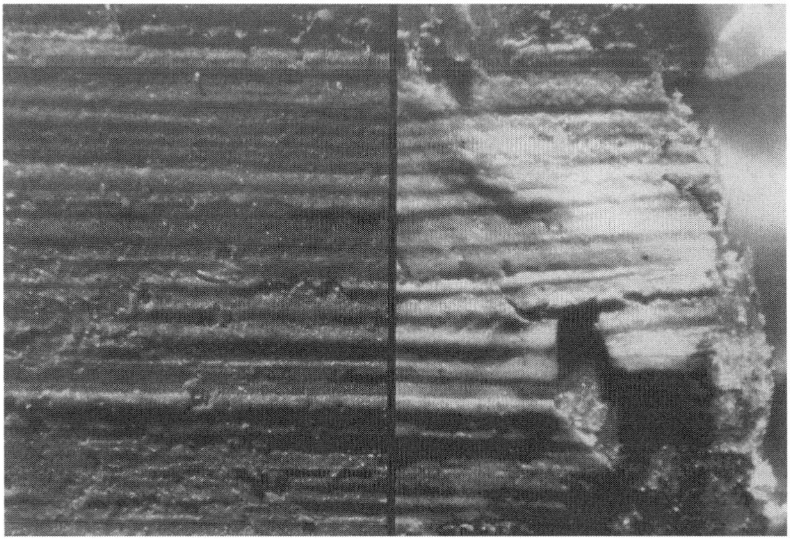

Figure 8.10 Comparison of replica cast of grinding on the surface of a tool (left) compared with a cast of the reverse of a fragment of paint (right).

fitted together. Clearly one of the most important aspects is the interpretation by the scientist of what detail is present, how it was formed and what level of variation may occur.

In general though, it should be fairly simple to provide a conclusive elimination if there are significant differences between the pieces and, given the type of examples of physical fits, such as those shown in Figures 8.1, 8.2 and 8.4, a conclusive link (or very strong level of support) would easily be possible. Given sufficient matching detail for a less than conclusive fit supported by manufacturing detail or for a contact fit, a conclusive link should still be possible.

However, where this falls short of the expert's threshold for their strongest level of evidence, a level of support can be given depending on how common they feel that type of item is (not forgetting that it may also be an uncommon occurrence to find that sort of item in pieces). In some cases, a direct physical fit examination involving comparison of fracture surfaces may not be possible. For example, the expert could be given pieces of a broken necklace where a chain link has been pulled and opened (rather than the metal itself being fractured) or pieces of the same item where an integral connecting piece is missing. However, a marks' expert may still be able to offer some level of support for the view that the pieces were once part of the same original item, based on any corresponding physical features that they may have. In this latter instance, a manufacturing marks' comparison would potentially be required, if possible.

9
Plastic Film Examinations

9.1 Introduction

A wide range of everyday objects are made from an equally large variety
of different plastics, with various methods available for their production.
One such method is the production of extruded plastic items, such as plastic
bags, sacks, wrappings, packaging materials and self-adhesive tape, using the
'blown film' process. This is where long lengths of plastic film are produced,
then cut or otherwise fashioned to make the desired product. Various marks
and other physical features from their production, which we shall describe,
may be present on these items and so they lend themselves well to forensic
examination and comparison. The general principles we have already seen
applied to tool marks are readily applied here.

In a forensic context, these items are commonly used for their intended
purpose, but with criminal intent, for example, they are used to wrap something, as in the case of packaging materials, or to stick something together, as
with self-adhesive tape. Packaging materials are commonly associated with
drugs; however, they can be used in many other types of case too, including
the disposal of human remains. Self-adhesive tape could also be used in
a number of circumstances, including, for example, terrorist cases for con-
structing incendiary devices, or kidnap where a victim is bound and gagged.
Reference (control or known) items could include, depending on the type of
item involved, single items, lengths of items joined together or whole rolls or
retail packets.

The questions that are generally being asked of this type of evidence relate
to establishing the source of the scene item, as with tool marks, but can
have additional evaluative issues relating specifically to how the items were
made and how one might expect the detail seen to change and alter with time.

The Forensic Examination and Interpretation of Tool Marks, First Edition.
David Baldwin, John Birkett, Owen Facey and Gilleon Rabey.
© 2013 John Wiley & Sons, Ltd. Published 2013 by John Wiley & Sons, Ltd.

Typical prosecution style questions include 'Is there any evidence to link these items?' or 'Are the scene and suspect item from the same common source?' However, in some instances, in order to do this, it may be necessary to try to place items in their sequential order of production or make a judgement on how well they correspond if no specific link is found.

In all cases, initially it will need to be established whether or not submitted items are of the same general type based on class features such as colour, size, construction and general appearance. If there is some level of agreement, then a more detailed examination may be carried out. Where there is no general agreement, the comparison would normally end. Aspects of initial and detailed examination with respect to particular types of blown film items will be discussed later in this chapter.

Another area of examination is that of physical fits of torn or cut blown film items. Essentially the techniques used to carry out a comparison can be applied to the examination of items to establish if they form a physical fit (Figure 9.1). If, for example, the marks' examiner can show that bags were sequentially manufactured, then this in itself is a form of physical fit. It is still a comparison of the torn or cut profile and using the detail produced during manufacture to confirm that items do or do not fit together.

As with other areas of marks' examination, the role of the crime scene examiner is critical in the success of the comparison of plastic film items. It is the ability to recover all of the relevant material that provides the opportunity to assess the rate of change in the detail. It is often the case where plastic bags are concerned that the suspect bag does not come from the top of a pile of

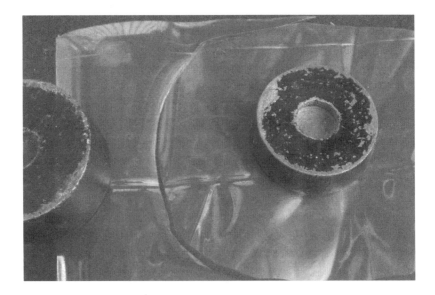

Figure 9.1   Physical fit of cut plastic film items.

bags but may come from somewhere in the pile. It is always best to remember that more recovered bags, film or tape is better than not enough.

9.2 The 'blown film' process

9.2.1 Extrusion

In a typical system for producing blown film (Figure 9.2), the plastic is heated until molten and then forced into the base of an upright cylindrical blowing machine. The liquid plastic passes up through a circular die (known as an 'annulus' or 'annular die'), which produces a tubular bubble of plastic. This part of the process produces what is known in forensic science as 'extrusion detail' in the plastic, which is a series of bands that run parallel to the direction of production. This extrusion detail can be fairly easy to see in

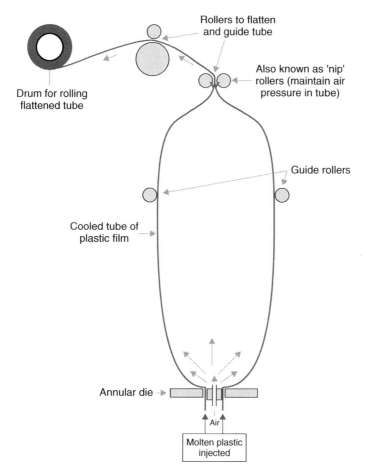

Figure 9.2 A typical system for producing blown film, for scale this would span three floors of a factory.

opaque, coloured plastics, but specialist lighting techniques will be necessary to visualise it in transparent plastics.

The bands are a result of the flow characteristics of the plastic through the annulus and can be affected by the position of the annulus, together with the build-up of solid waste plastic on its outside during use. Therefore, the extrusion detail can vary along the length of the plastic bubble, as there will be different and changing imperfections introduced at this point. The rate of change of the extrusion detail can be an important factor to take into consideration in any subsequent examination and evaluation.

The bubble then expands due to the air pressure maintained inside it. Any small imperfections in the plastic film in the region of the annulus will be magnified as the bubble expands. The solid waste is one of the possible reasons for the bubble to burst, which happens at intervals. When the bubble bursts, it is simpler to replace the annulus than to try to clean it *in situ*. Collars surrounding the cylinder partly act to both stabilise the bubble and cool the plastic, so that it is solid by the time it reaches the top of the cylinder. At the top, the blown film passes into a triangular array of rollers, which collapse the film into a double thickness sheet. The rollers can produce fine scratches on the surface of the plastic due to defects on their surfaces. Such scratches may also be introduced at other stages of manufacture and can change along the length of the plastic, sometimes within millimetres.

The system is very flexible; the thickness of the film can be controlled by the pressure of the air in the cylinder and by the speed of pulling, together with the rate of supply of the molten plastic to the annulus. Depending on the raw material used it is possible to produce clear/transparent plastics, coloured/pigmented plastics or to co-extrude two plastics through the annulus to give a two or more layered film with properties beyond those of a film made from a single material. There are different methods employed to achieve the colour required. Dyes can be used or in the case of black bin bags, carbon may be added. If solid pigment is added, as in the latter case, this may result in spots of pigment being left in the plastic, which can be visualised during laboratory examination.

It is also possible to introduce the 'male' and 'female' parts of a press/grip seal or zip seal into the bag construction during this initial extrusion phase. Another variation allows a textured surface to be formed on one side of the sheet, which is essential for retaining the adhesive on the plastic backing used for self-adhesive tapes. This is known as a 'tie coat', which leaves a backing pattern that the adhesive adheres to. A 'release coat' is applied to the top surface, which enables you to peel the tape rather than it sticking together permanently.

The tube of film is laid flat and nearly always split into suitable lengths before further processing into bags or other items. The double-thickness film may be slit lengthways to produce a pair of single-thickness sheets for other

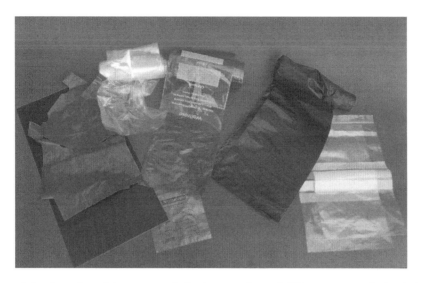

Figure 9.3 Examples of just some of the large variety of different types of plastic bags available.

purposes. The film is then rolled and transported for further processing into the desired product at the same, or a different, factory. Adhesive tape is made in long rolls, which can be cut to the correct width. Sometimes, these may be cut at an angle, meaning that there will be discrete orientation of the extrusion detail with respect to the edge of the tape (rather than it being exactly parallel to the edge).

9.2.2   Bag production and construction

There are a large variety of plastic bags available, which can show differences in their colour, size, general appearance and construction. Examples of just some of the types of bag are shown in Figure 9.3. All of these parameters can be used as discriminating features in a forensic examination and, therefore, require further explanation.

The production of bags from blown film can involve shaping the film, stamping out handles, forming gussets (a 'V' shaped fold at a side seam), heat sealing and perforating edges. In some cases a writing strip or printing is applied to the surface of the bag. The bags may also be given a surface texture by fine dimples being rolled onto the film. The key point here, however, is that the individual items are produced in sequence from a continuous sheet, and the processing maintains that order even to the point where the items are packed for retail sales.

9.2.2.1   Heat sealing, perforating and cutting There are many variations in the production methods used to convert the plastic tube into bags; some examples of the procedures involved will be given here (Plate 9). The simplest way of converting the plastic tube into bags is by heat sealing across it, and cutting the tube adjacent to this seal. This produces bags with a heat seal just above the bottom of the bag. If the bags are perforated rather than cut, the result is a continuous strip of joined bags, which may be wound into rolls. These can be torn off as necessary for use. If the tube is slit into two by a blade and then each half is heat sealed across the width of the blown tube, the original edges of the blown tube form the bottoms of two sets of opposed bags, with heat-sealed sides. If, however, a 'hot-knife' is used to split the tube into two or more sections, this effectively seals as it cuts. The tube can then be sealed across its width and cut/perforated as before, producing two or more parallel 'streams' of bags along the machine direction. Castle *et al.* (1994) gives more detail about the production and comparison techniques used for transparent plastic bags and wrapping film.

There are normally variations in the exact sizes of bags during a production run, largely as a result of fluctuations in the air pressure blowing the film. Therefore, only gross differences in size should be used to differentiate between bags. The position(s) of heat seals on a bag will often serve to give a reliable indicator of the machine direction and of the method of conversion of the blown film into the bag. The size and location of the heat seal can vary and the appearance of the heat seal can be useful, as it will sometimes show damage features that represent worn areas on the equipment. The presence of perforations at the top and bottom of a bag shows that the bag was derived from a roll of bags, with each bag being capable of being torn away from its neighbours on the roll. Although the tearing process potentially produces unique detail, stretching and distortion of the plastic attachment points frequently occurs, so that a true total physical fit between the two neighbouring bags cannot normally be demonstrated (although there may be some correlation of detail). Examples of a heat seal with intact and separated perforations are shown in Figure 9.4.

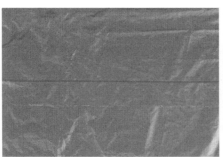 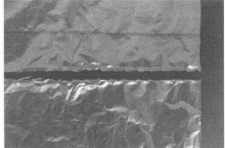

Figure 9.4 Examples of a heat seal with intact perforations (left) and separated perforations (right).

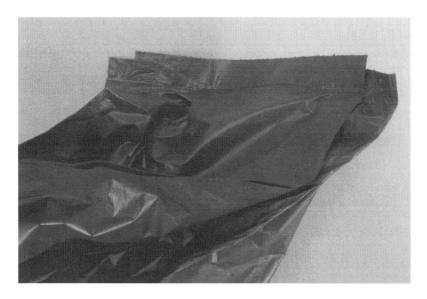

Figure 9.5   A side gusset on a bin bag, heat sealed at the bottom of the bag.

9.2.2.2   Gussets   Side gussets, which serve to enable a bag to be opened out at the top to a greater extent than the (generally) heat-sealed bottom, frequently occur in carrier bags and bin sacks. Some larger carrier bags have bottom gussets, which enable them to hold large items at the base of the bag. The plastic film can be folded to form the gussets, which are secured in place, usually by heat sealing (Figure 9.5). Small asymmetries are often seen in the alignment of the folds of the gusset, although there may be variation in the asymmetry between the top and bottom of a single bag.

9.2.2.3   Press seals   The components of this type of seal, also known as 'grip' seals, can be formed during the extrusion process (Figure 9.6) or can be heat sealed into the bag as a separate process. They consist of a 'male' part, in cross-section generally shaped like a mushroom, and a 'female' receptor in which the male part locates. Some bags of this type have a 'zipper' to enable the two parts of the seal to be closed or opened. Some otherwise colourless bags could have coloured grip seals, consisting of one or two colours.

9.2.2.4   Printing   This may take the form of text, along with white stripes or panels, intended to be written on by the user, to record the contents of the bags (Figure 9.7). These sometimes show small defects from the printing roller, which re-occur with every turn of the roller. There are occasions where there is more than one printing roller and alternate bags may be printed by the roller. Depending on the process, the print may occur in exactly the same place on all bags, but there are situations where the circumference of the roller does not correspond to an exact number of bags, causing the printing

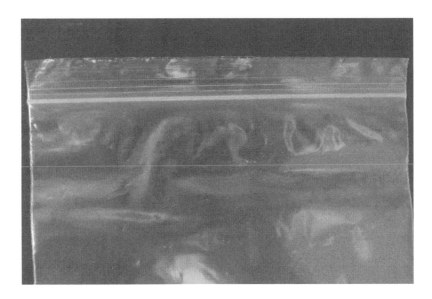

Figure 9.6   A press seal.

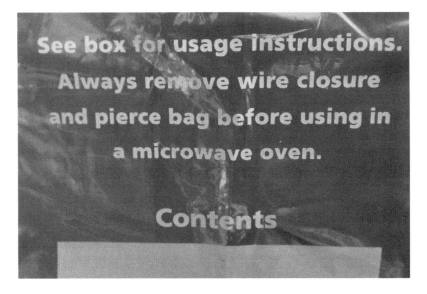

Figure 9.7   Printed text and white panel on a bag.

to be progressively displaced through the printing run, and any defective area to change position. This displacement of printing detail, particularly on perforated rolls of, for example, freezer bags, can be of use in establishing or eliminating potential physical fits and in the sequencing of such bags. Other forms of printing occur on many carrier bags, and the continuation of such printing across a 'join' is useful in confirming physical fits.

9.3 Laboratory considerations

While the general principles of marks' examination can be applied to the laboratory examination of plastic film items, it should be noted that these items can be recovered in very different sorts of offences from routine tool mark examinations, can involve large items and also the use of specialised equipment to visualise the production detail. Therefore, before we discuss the laboratory examination of items, additional considerations will be outlined here.

9.3.1 Preliminaries

The preliminaries required for this type of examination are very similar to those detailed in Chapter 4 for tool mark examinations. However, in these cases it is even more necessary to have a good idea of the background of the case and the expectations of the submitting officer.

In particular, the expectations can be well beyond what is achievable by an examination of the type of item being submitted, and it may be necessary to discuss the limitations with the investigating officer to ensure that the examination is still necessary. In drugs' cases, there may be occasions when a full detailed comparison of the plastic is not required as the drug's profile together with other evidence may be sufficient for the investigation.

Knowing the expectations, the examination can be planned. It is common in these cases that an examination for fingerprints or biological material requiring DNA analysis will be necessary and so examinations will often be multidisciplinary. These require good communication between the scientists involved to ensure that the items are examined in the correct order, and, where possible, that each evidence type is uncompromised by preceding examinations. Always check whether the tests involved will leave the plastic film in a fit condition for the marks' examination. Some fingerprint treatments, such as metal deposition or Ninhydrin, will stain and distort the plastic and therefore make it very difficult, if not impossible, to do a comparison. It may be possible to carry out a visual examination, prior to any treatment. It is important that Health and Safety and anti-contamination procedures are followed, as items may have been associated with, for example, drugs, body parts or chemicals from fingerprint treatments.

The laboratory space for the examination needs to be carefully considered; some of the equipment for plastic film examination is difficult to move very readily and it is best to conduct the examination as close as is practical to the equipment. Owing to the size of some bags the examination bench should, where possible, be of a sufficient size to accommodate the largest item when spread out; six average sized black dustbin bags occupy over $3\,m^2$ when spread out.

Collect and record the collection of the items; recording the collection is particularly important if they are being received from another scientist after their examination. It is also useful to check the condition of the items at that time. The individual plastic items should be labelled to make detailing the examination easier and to prevent confusing items that will have to be examined side by side.

If the submitted plastic items need to be examined for other forensic material, it is very important that details are known about the original condition. An example would be if layers of tape have been separated from each other, or an item cut apart. It is important that the original condition and sequence is known.

9.3.2 Equipment

In order to clearly visualise the extrusion detail in plastics, it is necessary to be able to transmit light through it. Generally speaking, a light box or table is useful for examining coloured/pigmented plastics, whereas specialised optical techniques, as described below, are required for transparent plastics. Under ordinary lighting conditions, transparent plastic appears to be just that, although it may be possible to visualise some detail under daylight by holding the plastic up to a window. One technique that is very useful in visualising and enhancing the extrusion detail requires the use of polarised light, which can be done using a piece of specialised equipment called a polarisation table in forensic science, although it may be called a strain gauge commercially. A typical set up is demonstrated in Figure 9.8.

Using this piece of equipment, a set of coloured extruded bands can be seen in some transparent plastics. This is as a result of the property known as 'birefringence'. This is because plastic that has been extruded will vary in its properties and thickness lengthways, along the direction of pull, compared with perpendicular to this direction. This can affect the way light travels through different parts of the plastic, as determined by its properties and thickness. When an item for examination is placed on the polarisation table, the light from the source underneath travels through a polariser, which makes all the light waves travel in the same direction. These light waves in turn travel through the item, interacting in a variety of ways to give different components of light, which are slightly rotated. As they exit the item, interference occurs between the out of phase light waves, and it is this interference that enables us to visualise the extrusion detail with the aid of the analyser.

Generally, polarisation colours are pale, low order greys with bands oriented in the direction the film was produced (Figure 9.9). For simplicity, we have only described plane polarisation here, which means that the

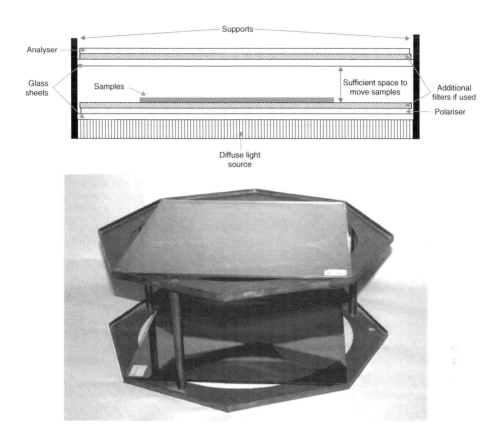

Figure 9.8 A diagram of a typical polarisation table, with an example of a very basic set-up for examining small bags shown underneath it.

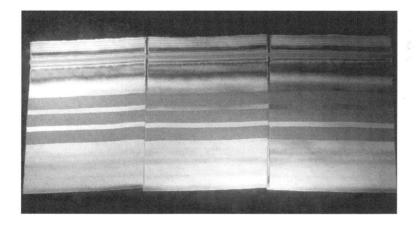

Figure 9.9 Low order grey polarisation colours, as seen using plane polarised light.

extrusion detail is only visible for certain orientations of the plastic film. However, other filters and analysers can be optionally introduced into the system, for example to allow the bags to be placed in any direction and still show banding, or to make the colours more vivid oranges and blues (Plate 10). This latter technique may used to improve the contrast of thin or weakly birefringent materials.

Another technique that can be used to visualise extrusion detail in transparent plastics is using a piece of specialised equipment known as a 'shadowgraph'. The shadowgraph comprises a narrow or parallel beam of light with the sample some distance from the source of parallel light. A screen is placed at a convenient point, not too far from the sample, to receive the image. Extruded detail will be visualised as a series of dark and light lines, which represent the differences in how the light passes through from the bulk material. This system can visualise very small changes in refractive index in a material. Whilst this piece of equipment is not commonly available commercially, one would be relatively easy to construct; an old-fashioned slide projector can be used as a light source (see Settles, 2001).

Other aspects of an examination can include comparison of heat seals, perforations and scratch detail on the surface of the plastic. With each of these areas an initial visual examination with your eye or with a low power bench microscope will provide some information, but eventually a specialist microscope is normally necessary. There are various microscopes that are very useful for this, with transmitted and reflective light sources which can be used by an examiner to view different microscopic features as necessary. Heavily pigmented plastics may not allow transmission of light and so it may not be possible to examine the extrusion detail. However, a microscopic examination of scratches and other surface detail can be carried out.

9.4   Laboratory examination and evaluation

Since there are many types of item made from blown film, only four sets of items that utilise blown plastic film in their construction will be considered here, as these are the most commonly encountered in a forensic context. These are:

- pigmented bags, such as rubbish bin bags and plastic carrier bags;

- transparent bags, such as self-seal bags;

- wrapping film, for example Cling Film™;

- self-adhesive tapes.

The techniques used for their examination cover most situations and can be generalised, as needed, to other items where thin blown plastic film has been used in their construction.

9.4.1   Pigmented bags

Pigmented bags, such as rubbish bin bags and plastic carrier bags, are those that have a colour to them and are generally opaque. There may be one or more questioned bags but, when possible, it is best to have a number of known bags for reference purposes. For simplicity, we will consider complete bags and first look at two bags for comparison, then an unknown bag (or bags) versus a known roll of bags, as this should highlight the comparison process, which would be similar for all categories of items considered here, followed by the difficulties that can be encountered in interpretation and evaluation.

9.4.1.1   One unknown bag versus one known bag   The type of question that is likely to be considered in this case is of the form 'Is there any evidence to link these bags?' or 'Are these two bags from the same source?' or maybe 'Did the two bags come from the same retail package?'
   Features that will be compared in the initial examination are:

- Colour and general appearance.

- Dimensions, that is the overall size, again only gross differences in size should be a discriminating factor.

- Method of construction, such as heat seals, perforations, gussets and printing on the bags. In particular, note the number of heat seals present. The heat seal at the bottom is particularly important as it usually wider than the others and will be a fixed distance from the top and bottom of the bag. For large bags note how the gusset is formed and its dimensions. If the items are from a tear-off roll, check that the perforations on the questioned bag are the same type as for the known bag.

- Other features such as:

  — Creasing, where bags have been folded, for example, carrier bags into a retail package.

  — Defects to cut edges and perforations.

The order in which the features are examined will depend on an assessment of the material being examined and deciding which features show most character or have most discriminating power. The expert will decide what features to compare and in which order. If significant differences are found, then the bags may have been made on different equipment and the examiner may terminate the examination. Another scenario where visual differences can occur is where the bags were produced on the same equipment, but not sequentially, so the detail caused by the production process has changed. Depending on the level of differences, the examination may be continued or terminated, as in this instance there are no other reference bags with which to assess the rate of change. Where there is correspondence in the above parameters, or it has been decided to carry out further work to determine either way, further more detailed examination could be carried out.

A comparison of extrusion detail would then follow. This is often best undertaken with the bag slit open, keeping the same orientation for each bag, so that they can be examined as single sheets. When cutting the bag open it is very important to do this very carefully and to cut away from other potential significant detail, such as printing or heat seals, as they may need to be examined further. Large bags will need a light table for the examination of the extruded lines/bands, but a light box may be sufficient for smaller bags. The banding of the two bags can be compared. Bands can be lighter or darker, narrower or broader, as shown in Figure 9.10, and so can be compared line by line. It may also have a very complex appearance where there are no discrete bands but the pigment pattern is almost herringbone in structure. Pigment particles may also be present and these could have a characteristic appearance under a microscope.

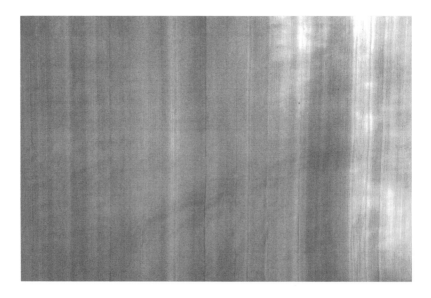

Figure 9.10 Extrusion detail of a bin bag, using transmitted light.

If two bags have been produced consecutively, then the extrusion detail will match and it should be possible to follow all the macro and micro features across the cut or perforated ends. If the bags have been made on the same production line and within a short distance of each other, the degree of agreement in the extrusion detail will depend on the rate of change of the extrusion detail. Clearly, the only way to assess this is to see how the detail changes over each of the bags. There will also be an expectation that the detail during a production run will change, so it may be that the reporting scientist may only be able to say that the bags were produced on the same production run but the differences are such that they are not from the same retail package. If the detail is very different in its appearance then it is only logical to say that the bags can be reported as being from different sources.

The amount of additional work that is required will depend on what degree of agreement is found with the extrusion detail and how characteristic is it. It is always worth looking at any plastic bags or film under a microscope using different light sources. In pigmented bags there may be features within the extrusion detail along the cut or perforated edge. For example, some particles have what is known as a 'fish tail' and if the particles/tails have been cut or perforated through, then they could line up in the correct position to confirm a fit. Other features could include creases in the plastic, irregularly cut edges and there may be extrusion features that travel across the edges at an angle.

If necessary, another examination that can be carried out between the two bags is looking at scratch detail running over the join where the two bags were potentially linked together. This detail can be visualised by using oblique reflected light. There may also be surface features in addition to scratches, which again may be very helpful. The scratches can be very short lived, change rapidly, are potentially randomly produced, be at angles to the cut ends and are often present all around the circumference of a bag. If there is a sufficient amount of characteristic scratch detail that matches and crosses the join, it may be the reporting scientist's opinion that there is a conclusive link between the bags.

It is not often the case that the bags are conclusively linked and in these situations it is useful to not only consider extrusion detail and scratches but also heats seals and printing if they are present, as they can add significantly to the findings. Matching microscopic irregularities in the heat seals will add to evidence that they were produced on the same production equipment.

9.4.1.2 Unknown bag(s) versus a roll/set of known bags The question that is often asked in this situation relates to establishing a link between the bags and showing that they are from a common source or specifically from a single retail package. The initial examination can proceed as for single bags, and where there are no significant differences, the comparison parameters may

help the examiner to discriminate and group bags where a number have been submitted.

Check the known bags first to determine which are the least variable extruded lines and their relationship to a given edge of the bag. Check that these bands are present in the questioned bag(s). If they are not all present, then the questioned bag(s) could have been made in the same run as the known bags but not at the same point. Clearly if there is a significant difference between the suspect bags and the control bags and the variation within the control population is limited, the evidence would suggest that the suspect bag or bags were not linked or that the link is limited. If the detail is completely different then the evidence clearly supports an alternative source.

Individual bags are formed and normally retained in sequence from a continuous sheet of plastic. Variation in the extrusion detail along the length of the sheet can occur but this will depend on the rate of change of the detail during the manufacturing process. Where the examination requirement is to connect a questioned bag (or bags) with a known roll or set of bags, the questioned bag should show banding that fits into the sequence of the known roll or set. If the bag(s) fits into the sequence of bags then this provides conclusive evidence of the bags originating from the known bags. If a single bag is considered, which fits at the end of a set of bags or a roll, we are always left with the possibility that this bag could have come from that roll or is the first bag on another roll or set of bags.

Sometimes, it may not be possible to sequence the questioned and reference bags. However, when a number of known bags are available, the variation in the extrusion detail can be observed by examining and comparing the first and last bags and possibly some bags at intervals in between, depending on how long a roll or set has been submitted. Some extruded bands may be long lived, appearing all the way through the roll; however, some may be more variable, appearing and disappearing over a relatively short length. A judgement can then be made as to whether the variation between questioned and known bags are what would be expected if they came from the same roll.

If all the long lived extruded lines are present, check the correspondence between the more variable bands in the two bags, and if there is good agreement then there is very strong evidence that the two bags were consecutively produced. If there is only a level of correspondence, look in the known sequence of bags for a bag with a similar proportion of long lived bands and variable bands. If one can be found, then this gives some indication of how far away the questioned bag could be from the closest matching bag in the sequence. With this information, together with some knowledge of how many bags were in the original retail pack, the evidence comes in the range of moderate to very strong, as we are trying to answer the question: 'Given the degree of matching detail, what is the likelihood that the bags are associated or is the degree of agreement just a chance occurrence?'

If the variable banding in the questioned bag lies outside the range in the known sequence or there are very few known bags available, then the evaluation becomes difficult. Clearly, if there is a degree of correspondence in the banding it will have some value, albeit limited. However, bags of all types are manufactured in vast numbers and without knowledge of the rate of change of the extrusion banding and other manufacturing detail that may be present, it is typical that the evidence lies between limited to moderate support that the bags came from the same retail pack.

A different situation arises when the all the extruded bands are long lived so that there is little variation in the known sequence of bags. In this case the questioned bag will either have extruded detail which closely matches that of the known sequence or it will not. However if there is no close agreement then the evidence is at best limited/moderate and it could be, depending on other information available, that there is no evidence to connect the bags. Even if there is a close match it does not necessarily show that the bags came from the same retail pack.

9.4.2 Self-seal bags

Cases involving drugs are frequently where self-seal bags are encountered. The questions are often regarding determining whether or not bags that contain drugs came from bags at a location thought to be involved in the packaging of the drug, or with other packages of drugs that may be found in the possession of a suspect.

Self-seal bags come in a variety of sizes, from small (around 50×70 mm in size) to larger A4 size. The larger bags often use a zipper style of closure, whereas the smaller use a 'push fit'. The shape of the tongue that fits into the groove varies between manufacturers, but the shape does not provide any great discrimination. It is normally the smaller bags that are sent for examination as they can be used to pack small quantities of illegal drugs. A common scenario is that a number of packs have been recovered from different individual users and it is required to connect these to the person who is suspected of supplying the drugs.

Firstly, check the dimensions and construction of the bags, noting especially the heat seals. Because the bags are usually small, there is a tendency to measure the bags too accurately. The machinery employed for their manufacture will allow a size variation of 0.5–1.0 mm and differences in that range can be ignored. Some bags have opaque strips for writing on printed on them; their dimensions and spacing are useful characteristic features, although their placement on the bag can be variable.

Secondly, if the bags all have the same class features, check the extrusion detail using a polarisation table. A rough check can be made using the bags as received but for a more detailed examination the bags need to be slit open

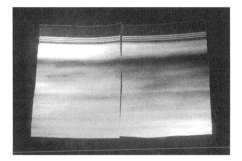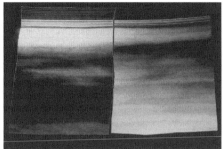

Figure 9.11   Single self-seal bag comparisons, showing a correspondence (left) and difference (right) of extrusion detail, which in this case has been visualised by polarisation, giving rise to polarisation colours.

down one side and at the bottom, so that it becomes a single sheet. Although the colours of the bands are important, the dimensions and relative positions of the bands are the main features used for matching.

The interpretation of the extrusion detail follows a similar line to that for pigmented bags. The main difference is that most self-seal bags are small so that there is not much variation in the lines along the bag's length (Figure 9.11). This can make placing the bags in sequence of production more complicated than for the pigmented bags. The evaluation of the findings is the same as for the pigmented bags.

9.4.3   Wrapping film

Plastic film is encountered in many cases, including drugs and firearms. The question is usually one of assessing whether or not the plastic wrapping came from a particular roll of film.

Wrapping film, sometimes called Cling Film™ in the United Kingdom, while made by the blown film process, is thinner and more heavily plasticised than the previous films. This affects the examination in two ways: the film distorts easily, especially when being torn, and the film normally produces diffuse pale grey colours when examined on the polarisation table. The shadowgraph will show flow and pull irregularities formed in the plastic during production, which results in differences in the way light travels through the film. There are two grades of wrapping film, domestic, which is clear, and catering, which is sold in longer rolls and is coloured.

The recovered film usually comes in one of three forms:

- Very long lengths, sometimes a complete roll, used for wrapping bulk items.

- Short lengths, under 1 m long, used for small quantities of material.

- Small pieces, used for wrapping individual doses of illegal drugs, which may have been in an offender's body orifice or travelled through their body and often require a DNA examination. The initial examination is unlikely to provide much useful information, being restricted to general appearance and sometimes to the width of the film.

Short lengths are normally the easiest to deal with. Often they have simply been torn from the roll of film and there can be a correspondence to the torn edge of the known roll of film. This will nearly always need confirmation by visualising the lines crossing the tear, using the shadowgraph. Long lengths provide practical problems. The materials being wrapped are typically of more importance to the investigating officer than the wrapping, so the film is often cut through to get to it. Unless the original external free end or internal free end can be unambiguously identified, a marks' examination is not justified. If the free ends have been preserved, then they can be compared with the free end of the known roll, by examining the shapes of the severed ends and using the shadowgraph to confirm any correspondence.

Small pieces of wrapping film that have been used to wrap drugs are difficult to examine. The film is usually tightly twisted around the drug and then knotted. It may also be heated and then sealed by melting the plastic. This process causes major distortions to the film, and if melted will mean that potentially a large section will be missing. In addition, the excess plastic film above the knot is often cut away so that no physical fit is possible either to other similar packs or to the original film. When opened out, the film has an approximately circular shape with a distorted dome profile, very often with traces of the contents ingrained in the plastic. Examination with the shadowgraph is not normally possible. If the excess plastic has not been cut away, the film will be more rectangular than circular although it will still have a dome profile. It may be possible to try to physically fit pieces back to other similar packs or to the original film. The creasing to the film normally prevents confirmation of the fit by using the shadowgraph.

In general, wrapping film will not be examined for scratch marks. As the film is so thin, scratches will normally result in tears rather than being left as surface detail. Other plastic films can be used for wrapping items, for example parts of plastic carrier bags. In these cases there is normally less distortion of the torn edges but confirmation of the physical fit may still be required. This can be done by examining the features that cross the tear, using the appropriate technique.

9.4.4 Self-adhesive tape

There are many types of tape encountered in various sorts of offence. Generally, the questions that are being asked relate to whether or not pieces of tape physically fit to a particular roll, or providing an opinion on whether or not tape came from a specific roll using manufacturing features. Ends of tape may be cut, or torn (using the fingers or mouth) and so often will be required for DNA and fingerprint examination. Fingerprints may be found on the top or back surface of the tape.

Two types of self-adhesive tape that are commonly encountered are general purpose clear tape, about 20–25 mm wide and brown packing tape, around 50 mm wide, although a range of widths are normally available for most tapes. Other types of tape may also be encountered, such as duct tape (or Duck Tape™), electrical insulating tape or patterned tape. The initial stage of the examination is to check that the known and questioned tapes have the same general appearance, surface texture, width and colour. Some latitude must be allowed in the colour matching if it is known that one of the items has been exposed to strong light or weathering but the other has not. Other parameters used could depend on the type of tape under examination. For example, duct tape has fabric strands forming a lattice through it, which could be counted and compared.

The detailed examination can take a number of forms. The requirement may be for very strong evidence that the crime and known tape were once joined. In that case a physical fit of the ends is the most likely technique to produce such a result (Figure 9.12). One method for doing this is to attach the ends to a sheet of clear material, such as a microscope slide or plastic sheet, so that they can be directly compared by overlaying them. Such a comparison is possible even when the ends have been cut, provided that the cut is not at right angles to the length of the tape. However, duct tape usually has a lot of irregularities and distortions, which will make this sort of comparison difficult. If the physical fit does not provide sufficient evidence, the ends can be microscopically examined in oblique reflected light for scratch marks crossing the ends.

It is also possible to remove the adhesive using a swab and solvent, but care is needed so that the solvent does not affect the plastic film. Sometimes,

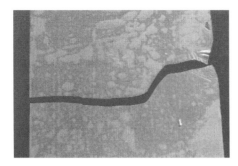 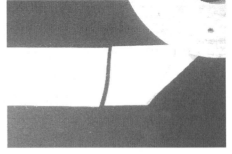

Figure 9.12   Physical fit comparison of torn brown tape (left) and cut electrical tape (right).

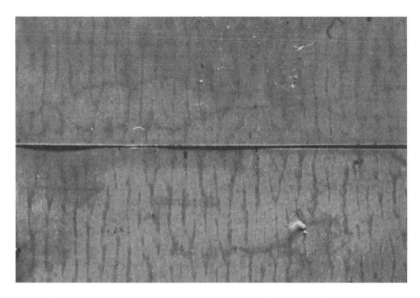

Figure 9.13 Backing pattern comparison of two pieces of tape. The free end of a roll of tape (top) and the end of a piece of tape cut from it (bottom).

for brown tape, it is the adhesive that provides the colour rather than the tape, and so after its removal, the tape will look clear. The plastic can then be examined on the polarisation table, which may on occasions appear black, thus indicating no polarisation effect. However, for some tape, polarisation colours are present but normally, due to the width of adhesive tape, there are usually insufficient bands for a detailed comparison. Removing the adhesive can also reveal the tie coat or backing pattern, which we discussed earlier. An example of two samples of tape corresponding in terms of their backing pattern is shown in Figure 9.13.

The figure shows the free end of a roll of tape (at the top) and the end of a piece of tape cut from it at the bottom. There is limited detail along the cut edges, but the backing pattern can be seen to cross the line between the pieces of tape, showing the separate piece originally came from the roll. If there is no physical fit then the backing pattern, which varies considerably in appearance, can show that tape has been produced on the same production line.

References

Castle, D.A., Gibbins, B. and Hamer, P.S. (1994) Physical methods for examining and vomparing transparent plastic bags and cling films. *Journal of the Forensic Science Society*, **34** (1), 61–68.

Settles, G.S. (2001) *Schlieren and Shadowgraph Techniques: Visualizing Phenomena in Transparent Media*, Springer-Verlag, Berlin, Heidelberg, New York.

10
Summary

This book has provided an overview of what the authors have, through personal experience, found to be a practical and successful approach to dealing with tool marks. The fundamentals of tool mark examination and comparison have been outlined, and we have sought to demonstrate how these principles can be applied to other related areas of work.

The area of forensic science covered is a very practical one. Visualisation of the detail present in a mark or on a bag or other item is one of the most important factors for interpretation and evaluation by the scientist. Clearly, this means that the 'pattern recognition' skills of an individual are very important, as this is a significant contributing factor to how quickly a person can identify the detail present and how successful they are in finding a 'match'. That is not to say that only certain people can do this area of work, although wry words may be whispered by experienced examiners of it being a 'black art' or 'a connoisseur's mark' when faced with a difficult examination. What this implies is that only examiners with a high level of expertise would be able to see the detail. We would disagree completely with this sentiment. It should be recognised that this is a subjective area of forensic science and there are many skills an individual can use, such as visualising and manipulating images in their head, which have little, if anything, to do with academic qualification and training. However, if individuals have the right training and coaching and use the appropriate equipment then they can become very competent examiners.

It is worth saying at this point that it should not be forgotten that the examination and comparison of firearms/ballistics can be considered to be a specific and specialist example of a tool mark examination. This has not been considered in this book, as there are many subtle and significant differences with the kind of examinations we have described. There has been considerable research and development work carried out in this field by scientists in the United States. The Association of Firearms and Tool Mark

The Forensic Examination and Interpretation of Tool Marks, First Edition.
David Baldwin, John Birkett, Owen Facey and Gilleon Rabey.
© 2013 John Wiley & Sons, Ltd. Published 2013 by John Wiley & Sons, Ltd.

Examiners (AFTE) continue to undertake very important research and is an excellent source of background information. Within the firearms and tool mark community in the United States, an attempt to introduce a method of assessing what constitutes a match for striation marks has long been a goal. The work of various examiners, and specifically Biasotti (1959, 1964, 1980), led to the development of an approach termed 'Consecutive Matching Striations' (CMS) (Bunch, 2000).

This is an approach, with an established set of rules, which attempts to remove some of the subjectivity in saying whether or not striations in a test mark and on a questioned item match. It was originally designed for comparison of striations on bullets, which have a restricted set of variables in how they are made, due to the way a bullet passes through a gun barrel. However, it has since been applied to three-dimensional striated marks as well. No such technique is available for comparing impressed marks, and so it has limited application in a wider sense, but is well worth reading about should you be interested.

Another keen area of research is the development of methods and equipment to undertake an initial automated comparison and to provide an objective measurement of any match. At present, these systems are a tool that can be used to assist the expert, by initially comparing marks and providing results that need to be verified by an examiner. As is often the way with automated systems, they are able to deal with good quality marks where the detail is clear and well defined but still encounter problems when there is lots of interference or the detail is poorly defined. In these cases, the eye is still often the best imaging system available. It is early days, but as software and user interfaces develop, improvements are likely to be made. Ahlhorn *et al.* (2000), Geradts *et al.* (2001), Augustyn *et al.* (2001) and Scott Chumbley (2010) are a few such papers that document the foray into this area of research.

In reading this book the authors hope that you have developed an understanding and appreciation of the subject and its complexities and a wish to investigate the subject more.

References

Ahlhorn, T., Katterwe, H., Braune, M., *et al.* (2000) Computerised comparison of tool-marks. *Information Bulletin for Shoeprint/Toolmark Examiners*, **6** (1), 29–37.

Augustyn, A., Kowalski, P., Luchowski, L., *et al.* (2001) Computer-assisted analysis of striated toolmarks and impressions. *Problems of Forensic Sciences*, **XLVII**, 291–299.

Biasotti, A.A. (1959) A statistical study of the individual characteristics of fired bullets. *Journal of Forensic Sciences*, **7** (1), 34–50.

Biasotti, A.A. (1964) The principles of evidence evaluation as applied to firearms and toolmark identification. *Journal of Forensic Sciences*, **9** (4), 428–432.

Biasotti, A.A. (1980) Firearms and toolmark identification – A forensic discipline. *AFTE Journal*, **12** (3), 12–15.

Bunch, S.G. (2000) Consecutive matching striations criteria: A General critique. *Journal of Forensic Sciences*, **45** (5), 955–962.

Geradts, Z., Zaal, D., Hardy, H., *et al.* (2001) Pilot investigation of automatic comparison of striation marks with structured light. *Proceedings of SPIE*, **4232**, 49–56.

Scott Chumbley, L. (2010) *Final Technical Report August 25, 2009: Quantification of Tool Marks*. Work conducted at Ames Laboratory, Iowa State University under the Department of Justice Interagency Agreement number 2004-R-IJ-088, M-003, dated September 2004.

Glossary

analyser a second polarisation filter that can be rotated relative to the first polarisation filter in optical equipment to visualise variations in the object being examined.

angle grinder also known as a *disc grinder*, this is a handheld power tool used for cutting, *grinding* and polishing.

anisotropic a physical property (such as *refractive index*) of an object that is directionally dependent, that is, it varies, when measured along different axes. One example of anisotropy is *birefringence* and this can be seen when viewing light passing through an object using a polariser.

annular die a *die* with a circular aperture through which material can be extruded. Of interest here is the *extrusion* of the blown plastic film to form bags or the *extrusion* of plastic coating for electrical wires.

anvil cutter a cutting tool, such as a pair of secateurs, that has one jaw with a flat plate against which the object to be cut is held while the sharpened blade on the other jaw cuts through it. It will normally leave an *impressed mark* on one side of the cut object and *striations* on the cut end that lead from only one side.

back mark a mark, usually in the form of an impression, made by part of a *levering tool* set back from the tip. It can be made by the blade or *shaft* of the tool and is normally the pivot point during the levering action.

ball pein hammer this type of hammer is designed for use by metal workers and engineers. One part of the head is normally flat and round and is used to drive in nails. The other (the ball pein) is dome shaped and is usually used to shape metal and close rivets.

band saw a type of *saw* where the teeth are *set* on a continuous band that rotates in one direction. The object to be sawn is usually fed across the blade.

The Forensic Examination and Interpretation of Tool Marks, First Edition.
David Baldwin, John Birkett, Owen Facey and Gilleon Rabey.
© 2013 John Wiley & Sons, Ltd. Published 2013 by John Wiley & Sons, Ltd.

beading a strip of material used to hold glazing in place in a door or window. On double glazing units it is usually made of plastic or metal that clips into place in the *frame*. On older wooden windows and doors it is usually a piece of shaped wood strip that is nailed in place.

bevel used to signify that the tip of a tool has been shaped, usually by *grinding*, at an angle to produce a sharpened tip.

bevelled edge primarily used to describe the edges of a tool (other than the tip) that have been partially angled, but not sharpened.

birefringence this is an optical property of a material with variations in *refractive index* that depends on the propagation direction of light. Such materials are optically *anisotropic*.

bolt croppers a tool with two cutting blades, originally designed to cut through metal bolts, but can be used to cut through materials of suitable size and thickness, such as *padlock shackles* and chain links.

bolt cutters the same as *bolt croppers*.

brick bolster a metal chisel with a wide blade.

cabinet screwdriver the blade on this type of *screwdriver* is effectively straight and parallel and meets the tip at a right angle. The blades of such *screwdrivers* are often produced by simply *grinding* the *faces* onto a metal rod.

cable cutter a double-bladed cutting tool designed for cutting through heavier duty cables. One blade is often partially concave to hold the cable and prevent it from being squeezed out of the jaws. Some commercial cutters for heavy duty cables have blades that are clamped around the object to be cut.

cable ties a plastic tie with a strap that passes through the head with a ratchet action to hold it tight. Most are single use, but some are designed so that the ratchet can be released and the tie used again. Also known as *ratchet ties* or *security ties*.

case opener a generic name often used for a variety of *levering tools*, including *wrecking bars*, crow bars, *pry bars*, and so on.

cast a mould taken (usually in silicone rubber) from a mark or a tool. It shows the detail of the object from which it was taken in reverse.

casting material material used to take a *cast* from an object. Silicone rubbers are normally used, but a polysulfide material may be used to make an intermediate in producing a *replica cast*.

centre meet cutters any form of cutting tool with two jaws, such as *bolt cutters*, *wire cutters* and *pliers*, with two cutting blades that meet together once the object has been cut through. The cut ends will have *striations* on them leading from both sides, with possibly impressions of the *cutting edges* of the blades in the central portion of the cut end.

chisel blade normally used to describe the blade of a chisel, which is parallel sided with a bevelled (sharpened) *leading edge*. It can also be used to describe the flat bladed end of a *case opener* or similar tool.

circular saw a *saw* fitted with a blade that has teeth around the circumference, that operates with a rotating action.

class features also known as class 'characteristics'. These are features that have been determined prior to production of a particular tool, such as the type and action of the tool and its size and general shape. Many tools will have the same *class features*.

clawed end the split or forked part of the head of a *claw hammer* or one or two blades of a *case opener* or pry bar.

claw hammer a hammer on which the head has one part (usually round) for striking nails and the other is forked to allow nails to be pulled out.

close cut usually used in connection with *bolt cutters* where the blades are asymmetrical in cross-section allowing one side of the tool to cut very close to a surface, leaving only a very shallow projecting stump.

closing edge the edge of a door or window away from the hinged side that closes onto the *frame*. This is the part often attacked with a levering tool to force open the door/window.

club hammer this may also be known as a lump hammer. It has a double-faced head, and is normally used with *cold chisels* and for some demolition work. The head is usually square or octagonal, but can be shaped to give a round *face*.

cold chisel this tool is designed for cutting metals, but can also be used as a *levering tool*. They are forged to shape and hardened and tempered at the cutting edge. They come in a variety of sizes, from fine engraving tools to very large chisels that are used with a sledgehammer.

comparator a specialist microscope with a single set of eyepieces mounted on a bridge fitted with two sets of objective lenses, to view two different objects simultaneously. In *tool mark* examinations these are usually the crime and *test marks*. This equipment may also be known as a *comparison macroscope* or *comparison microscope*.

comparator stage a stage on a *comparator* onto which objects are mounted to be viewed under the objective lenses. They are normally made to be moved smoothly in three dimensions and to be tilted at different angles.

comparison macroscope an alternative name for a *comparator* especially when low magnification macro objectives are used.

comparison microscope an alternative name for a *comparator*.

control item this is an item from a known source against which other items are compared. In tool mark cases it will be the tool itself and any *test marks* made with it. For *manufacturing mark* and *physical fit* cases it will usually be the items seized from a suspect or other known location that are to be compared with similar materials recovered from a scene of crime or from other locations to be linked back to the suspects.

crime mark a mark left at the scene of a crime. It can also be used to describe any *cast* of a mark, or marks on an item, recovered from the scene.

cross-head screwdriver a generic term used to describe a *screwdriver* where the head has been manufactured with four flutes at right angles. Specific brands using cross heads include Philips™ and Posidriv™.

cross pein hammer along with the *claw hammer*, this is a standard household hammer. One part of the head is round and is used to drive in nails. The other is flat and is usually at right angles to the handle (the cross pein). In the home, the pein can be used for starting to drive in small nails and tacks.

cutting edges the edges of a cutting tool that pass through the object being cut. They can be sharp as in *wire cutters*, scissors, knives and *cable cutters* or have flattened edges as in *bolt cutters* where the cutting is achieved by the pressure applied to the blades to force them through the material.

cutting mark a mark made by any type of cutting tool, including *saws*, knives, *bolt cutters* and *wire cutters*.

depth of field the vertical distance between where the highest and lowest features in the microscope image plane retain their image sharpness without the need to refocus.

diagonal cutters another name for *wire cutters* or *side cutters*, which have *centre meet cutting* jaws used for small diameter materials such as wires.

die a tool used to cut or shape material, such as plastic, to form an object. The shaping may occur when a *die* is used to extrude material.

disc cutter a cutting tool that uses discs to cut through an object with a rotary action. The discs are often made of metal with abrasive particles around the circumference, rather than being made entirely of abrasive material.

disc grinder a cutting tool that uses abrasive discs to grind material from an object or to cut through it.

double-bladed cutter any cutting tool that has two blades, such as *bolt cutters*, *cable cutters*, *wire cutters* and secateurs.

double-bladed end the blade of a tool (*case opener* or *claw hammer*) that has two prongs. Also known as a *forked end*.

duck tape another name for *duct tape*, deriving from the material originally used as the backing being duck cloth. Also a trade name for some tapes.

duct tape a self-adhesive/*pressure sensitive tape* with a cloth backing that is often coated with plastic of different colours. The adhesive can be of different types so that some tapes are permanent and others can be removed easily.

dynamic mark a mark produced when an implement slides across a surface. It is usually associated with a tip or edge of the implement making contact, but some *back marks* may contain apparent *grinding detail* that has been caused by the tool slipping to leave *striations* in the otherwise *impressed mark*.

end cutters a tool, such as *bolt cutters*, where the *cutting edges* are on the ends of the blades such that the tool is presented in line to the piece of rod or wire that is to be cut, rather than side on.

end impression an *impressed mark* left when a tool has slid along a surface and stopped. The angle that this impression makes to the plane of the *sliding marks* can be used to estimate the angle at which the tool was making contact with the surface.

extrusion this is a process where a material, such as plastic or metal is pushed or drawn through a *die* formed to the cross sectional profile of the object to be produced. It can be used to create objects of complex cross-sections.

extrusion detail detail produced on the surface of an object formed by *extrusion* by defects in the *die(s)* used.

face one side of the blade of a tool.

flash excess metal squeezed out between two *dies* during the *forging* process that does not break off leaving a ridge around the edge of the object produced in the *dies*.

foreshortening the effect caused by pulling a tool across a surface at an angle to the direction of movement. The width of the resultant marks is less than the width of the tool used. The greater the angular difference, the more *foreshortening* occurs.

forked end the blade of a tool (*case opener* or *claw hammer*) that has two prongs. Also known as a *double-bladed end*.

forging this is the process shaping of metal under the application of force. This was traditionally done by a blacksmith using a hammer and anvil to shape metal, but today powered machinery is often used to aid the operator or even automated machinery can be used with minimal operator input.

frame the fixed part of a door or window, against which or into which a tool may be pressed during forced entry. It is also the term for the main body of a *hacksaw* into which the blade is inserted.

glancing mark a mark made by an implement striking a surface at an angle and sliding across it rather than hitting it fairly square on. *Glancing marks* usually comprise *striations*, although there may be partial impressions at the end.

grinding a process of using an abrasive material, such as carborundum (silicon carbide), bound into a matrix to form *wheels*, discs or other more complex shapes to remove metal from a partially finished tool to erase imperfections, impart its final shape or to form a sharp cutting edge.

grinding detail when applied to tools this refers to the highly characteristic *striations* left on the *faces*, sides or edges of tools that have been ground during manufacture. It is also used as a generic term to include detail left on tools by a *linishing belt*, which is similar to *grinding detail*.

grinding disc/wheel a disc comprising abrasive particles held in a matrix to be used with an *angle grinder* or other mechanical *grinding* tool. The abrasive is constantly sacrificed during use and hence detail left on objects being ground will not be reproducible.

grip marks marks left on an object when held between the jaws of a *gripping tool* such as a vice, locking *pliers*, *wrench*, and so on.

gripping tool a tool with two jaws, which can be used to hold an object with one jaw on either side. Some, such as vices and locking *pliers*, are designed to be clamped onto the object but others, such as *pliers*, only grip the object while hand pressure is applied to the handles of the tool.

grip-seal bag a plastic bag that can be sealed by pressing together interlocking strips on the inner surfaces. It can be opened and resealed many times. Also known as a *press-seal* or *self-seal bag*.

hacksaw a *saw* formed with a 'U' shaped *frame* holding a removable blade 12 (or 10) inches long. The blade can be removed either to replace it when worn or damaged or to fit a blade with different properties.

hasp a fastening that is usually hinged and slotted to fit over a *staple* and can be secured by a *padlock* or pin.

hooked end the curved end of a *case opener* or *wrecking bar* that is usually forked and used to extract nails or to give better access between surfaces where the geometry precludes the use of a long, straight tool.

impact mark a mark formed when an implement has been used to hit a surface (such as a hammer blow).

impressed mark a mark formed when an implement is forced into a surface. This is often from a gripping or levering action, but *impressed marks* can also be found where dynamic marks come to an end or when a tool has impacted onto a surface (such as a hammer blow).

individual characteristics random detail that has been acquired during the manufacturing process or through use. This detail will not be reproduced on more than one item.

injection moulding a process for producing objects from plastic (or other materials). The material to be moulded is heated and forced (injected) into a mould cavity where it cools and hardens to form the required object. The moulds are usually made from metal and may have one or more cavities machined to form the features of the object to be produced.

insulating tape a form of pressure-sensitive tape that is normally used to insulate electrical wires. Such tapes are made of plastic, often vinyl because it stretches easily and has good insulating properties.

intermediate cast a *cast* made from either an original *cast* or an object, usually in a polysulfide compound, that is then recast to form a *replica cast*.

jaws of life an item of cutting equipment normally used by the emergency services for freeing victims from crushed vehicles. They are usually double-bladed cutting jaws operated hydraulically to give greater cutting power.

jemmy (US = jimmy) this is a term associated with *case opener*, crowbar, *wrecking bar* and *pry bar* type tools. It is usually used to refer to the tool when used for burglary.

junior hacksaw a small *hacksaw* taking blades 6 in long.

kerf the cut or groove left by a *saw*. It can also refer to the width of such a cut.

leading edge the edge of the tool that moves across or through a surface. For a *levering tool* this will usually be the tip and for a cutting tool it will usually be the cutting edge of the blade.

levering tool any tool that can be used to lever open a door, window or other object, whether designed for levering or not. Commonly encountered *levering tools* are *case openers* (and related tools) and *screwdrivers*, but almost any bladed implement can fall into this category.

light box/table a diffuse light source, formed into a box or table, for giving even illumination of an object from below.

linishing in the context of this book, *linishing* is a form of *grinding* using a continuous abrasive-coated belt rather than an abrasive wheel. It is normally used to flatten or smooth the surface of a tool. Technically, it can also refer to using increasingly fine grades of abrasive belts to prepare a raw metal object for final polishing.

linishing belt a continuous abrasive belt used to give a final shape or finish to a tool.

locking pliers *pliers* with adjustable jaws that can be clamped onto an object to hold it. The spacing of the jaws is *set* by a bolt in one of the handles.

lock striking plate usually attached to a door *frame*, this is the plate into which the bolt or tongue of a lock engages.

long working length strictly speaking this refers to a long working distance microscope objective, which is one designed to have longer free working space between the objective and the item than a normal objective of the same magnifying power.

manufacturing marks detail introduced onto the surface by the machinery or other processes during manufacture. Depending on the type of detail and how it was produced, this detail may appear on many other items produced with the same equipment or it may change rapidly, such that no two items have the same detail imparted on them.

match correspondence of impressed or striated detail between a *scene mark* and the tool being compared. Also, correspondence of characteristic profiles or surface characteristics for *physical fit* or *manufacturing mark* comparisons. Identifications are often referred to as 'matches'; however, the term is also used when *individual characteristics* correspond, even if the level of evidence is less than conclusive.

mechanical fit another name for a *physical fit*.

micron a unit of linear measurement, represented by the symbol μ. It is 1×10^{-6} m.

modus operandi **(MO)** the method of committing a crime, such as means of entry or actions taken by the offender.

monkey wrench: an adjustable *wrench* now used mainly for heavier tasks. It can be (mistakenly) used to refer to a *pipe wrench*.

moulage a French term for any moulding or *casting material* that was often used in early books of forensic science, but rarely used today. It now more often refers to materials used to simulate wounds on a person either for medical training or theatrical purposes.

multi-tool a small tool combining a variety of different attachments, which may include penknife blades, *screwdriver blades*, *pliers* and scissors among others.

padlock a portable lock that can be used in conjunction with a *hasp* and *staple*, chain or shutters to secure premises or property.

padlock shackle the moveable part of a *padlock*, often 'U' shaped, that is passed through a *staple* (of a *hasp* and *staple*) or two ends of a chain to secure them.

panel saw to the layman a *panel saw* is considered to be the standard hand *saw* used in woodworking and carpentry to cut pieces of wood to shape and size. This is usually done in order to join the pieces together and create a wooden object. The blade is usually fairly large with one edge having a series of sharp points or teeth to cut through the wood. A *panel saw* can also be a *circular saw* set in a bench used to cut large panels of wood into smaller pieces. They tend to have the fewest teeth per inch of all the commonly used *saws*.

physical fit the comparison of objects from two locations to see if they originated from a single item, by looking at characteristic profiles of the ends or features on the two items that continue on both sides of the break.

pincers a tool used to cut or pull an object such as a nail that has been hammered into a surface. *Pincers* have two jaws, perpendicular to the length of the tool, which are usually forged or ground to a relatively sharp edge. They can be brought close to the surface and closed around the nail to grip or cut through it. The curved shape of the jaws allows them to be pivoted around to pull out the nail, potentially leaving an *impressed mark* on the surface. Some *pincers* also have a small forked blade for use as a nail puller on the end of one of the handles.

pipe cutter a tool with at least one sharp wheel and an adjustable jaw used to grip and cut metal pipe. A *pipe cutter* is used by rotating it around the pipe and repeatedly tightening it until it has cut through the pipe completely. It produces a much cleaner cut than a *hacksaw*. Also known as a *tube cutter*.

pipe wrench a form of adjustable *gripping tool* designed for use on soft iron pipes and fittings with a rounded surface. The jaws have angled teeth that dig into the surface as the *wrench* is turned. Can also be known as Stilsons or *Stilson wrench* after the original inventor of this type of tool.

plane polarised light light is normally formed of waves vibrating in all directions. By passing it through a polarisation filter the wave train will then vibrate in a single direction. An example of the use of the polarisation of light is in some sunglasses, which reduce glare by cutting out light that has been reflected off a surface and thus tends to vibrate in one direction.

pliers a *gripping tool* with two pivoted arms The jaws that close on the item being gripped are usually serrated. They come in various shapes and sizes, some being long and thin, others being relatively short and blunt. As well as gripping, many *pliers* also have centre meet *cutting edges* and some even have a *scissor action* for cutting wires on the outside of the handles in the area around the pivot.

pressed detail detail impressed on the *face* of a tool such as a *screwdriver* when it is forged.

press-seal bag another term for a *grip-seal bag*.

pressure sensitive tape known variously as adhesive tape, self-adhesive tape or sticky tape. As its name suggests this type of tape sticks to another surface when pressure is applied, without having to moisten it or use solvent or heat. There are many uses for tapes of this type.

pry bar another term for the range of tools including *case opener*, crowbar, *wrecking bar* and so on.

questioned item an item, usually recovered from a scene of crime, that is to be compared with a tool or items from a known source to see if any links can be established.

ratchet ties another name for *cable ties*.

redressed dressing is a process by which stones, including *grinding* stones or wheels, are given smoother surfaces. As *grinding wheels* are used, the surfaces become worn and unsuitable for use; at this stage they are *redressed* to give them a smoother surface again.

refractive index a measure of the ratio of the speed of light in a vacuum to that in another medium.

replica cast a *cast* made using an intermediate that replicates an original *cast* or tool. May also be known as a 'recast'.

reflective light a light source, usually for microscopy, where the object being examined is illuminated from above and the light is reflected from it into the optics allowing surface features to be examined.

release coat a coating applied to the upper surface of a plastic film used for *pressure sensitive tapes*, so that the finished roll can be unwound without the layers sticking together.

relief coat another term occasionally used for a *release coat*.

retardation plate a sheet of optically active material that can be combined with polarising filters to produce specific optical path length differences, which increase the usefulness of polarised light in the examination of materials.

saw any tool with a toothed blade used to cut through an object. This includes *panel saws, tenon saws, hacksaws, band saws, circular saws*, and so on.

saw blade a toothed *saw blade* can be simply attached to a handle, as in panel and *tenon saws*, or inserted into a *frame* such as in *hacksaws*. More specialised blades are used in *circular saws*, where the teeth are arranged around the circumference of a circular blade, or *band saws* where the blade forms a continuous strip.

scene mark same as '*Crime mark*'.

scissor action relates to double-bladed cutting tools where, instead of the two blades meeting together, one blade passes over the other effectively shearing through the object being cut. There will be *striations* on both cut ends with those on one end coming from one side and those on the other coming from the opposite side. Scissors are an obvious example of this type of tool, which also includes *tin snips* and bypass secateurs and loppers.

scratches *striation* marks can also be referred to as *scratches* or scratch marks. *Scratches* are also random features introduced onto a tool when it scrapes against a hard object.

screwdriver this is clearly a tool used to insert or remove screws (and other threaded items such as bolts) by rotating them. It comprises a blade or head (the tip of which is placed in a screw head), with a *shaft* leading to a handle. *Screwdrivers* are made in a variety of shapes and sizes. In normal use the tip of the blade is inserted in the head of the screw and rotated. In criminal use *screwdrivers* can be used as levering tools to good effect.

screwdriver blade the part of a *screwdriver* that is inserted into a screw head. The two main forms are flat and cross-headed.

security ties another term for single use *cable ties*.

self-seal bag a plastic bag that can be sealed by pressing together interlocking strips on the inner surfaces. It can be opened and resealed many times. Also known as a *grip-seal bag*.

set arrangement of teeth on a *saw blade* to produce a *kerf* wider than the blade itself.

shaft on a *screwdriver* this is the part of the tool between the blade and the handle. On a *case opener* it is the part between the blades at either end.

side cutters this is another term that can be used for *diagonal cutters* or *wire cutters*, which have *centre meet cutting* jaws used for small diameter materials such as wires.

silanized paper paper with a coating on one side, normally applied so the paper can be used as a removable backing sheet for self-adhesive films. The treated surface will adhere to silicone rubbers while they are curing allowing them to be labelled.

sledge hammer designed for heavy tasks, such as breaking up concrete, stone or masonry, or to hammer in wooden posts, a *sledge hammer* can also be used to knock through a door. Because of its long handle a *sledge hammer* can be swung like an axe. The head is usually square or octagonal, but can be shaped to give a round *face*.

sliding mark a mark made when an object slips or slides across a surface. *Tool marks* made in this way normally comprise *striations*, although there may also be some impressed detail at the end of the *striations*.

slotted screwdriver a *screwdriver* used for screws that have a simple, straight slot cut across the head. This is the standard *screwdriver* for home use and can also be known as a flat or flat-bladed *screwdriver*.

staple the part of a security system over which a *hasp* is placed to be held in place with a *padlock* or pin. Also a 'U' shaped fixing used to hold sheets of paper together.

Stilson wrench a form of adjustable *gripping tool* designed for use on soft iron pipes and fittings with a rounded surface. The jaws have angled teeth that dig into the surface as the *wrench* is turned. Named after the original inventor of this type of tool.

striations/striae a series of ridges and grooves produced when a tool slides across a surface. They are formed by imperfections, often microscopic, along the edge of the tool making contact with the surface.

sub-class features features that are not unique to one particular item, but allow some discrimination between groups of tools with the same *class features*. They arise during manufacture, but are not necessarily introduced deliberately. The source of *sub-class features* may change over time.

submitting authority the *submitting authority* is the organisation that submits a case and requests the examination. It is usually the police, but can also be other agencies such as customs or defence lawyers. In some jurisdictions it may also be the investigating magistrates or courts.

swan neck on a *case opener* this is area of the *shaft* where it curves round at one end.

swarf small fragments of metal removed by a tool such a *saw* or a drill. Small lips of *swarf* may be left on a cut surface if the *saw blade* has stopped before it was completely removed.

tenon saw this is a *saw* with brass or steel on the back of the blade to stiffen it. The stiffness and extra weight allows more accurate, straight cuts to be made in small pieces of wood, the back of the *saw* restricts the depth of cut that can be made. Such a *saw* is best used to cut small pieces of wood and to form joints. They normally have around 10–14 teeth per inch.

test mark a mark made in the laboratory with a suspected implement. It can be made in a variety of materials to best reproduce the *scene mark*. The term can also be used for a *cast* made from such a mark.

tin snips these are scissor type cutters with long handles and short blades designed for cutting sheet metal. The main types of *tin snips* are used to make straight (or slightly curved) cuts, although there are others that can be used to cut tight curves or circles.

tip mark a mark left by the part of a tool blade close to the tip. Although normally associated with levering tools, *tip marks* can also be seen in some *cutting marks* where the object being cut has not been fully inserted between the cutting blades.

tip profile the shape of a tool tip of, which is often highly characteristic, especially if damaged or broken. The *tip profile* can be seen in *impressed marks* or is represented by the contact points in *sliding marks*.

tool mark a mark left by an object hitting or sliding across a surface. This is normally left by a tool, but any other object such as a ring, a domestic iron or even a vehicle can be considered as a 'tool'.

transmitted light a light source, for microscopy, where the object being examined is illuminated from below and the light passes through it, rather than being lit from above.

tube cutter an alternative name for a *pipe cutter*.

tyre lever (US = tire iron) a levering tool, often with at least one end having a blade with a rounded *tip profile*, but they are available in many shapes and sizes.

unique characteristics another term for *individual characteristics*.

utility bar another *case opener* type tool, usually with two *forked ends* and apparently made from a strip of metal rather than from a rod or hexagonal bar.

wire cutters *wire cutters* (also known as *diagonal cutters*) are normally used for cutting through wires or very small diameter materials. They have *centre meet cutting* blades on the jaws.

wood chisel *wood chisels* are designed to cut small amounts of wood and have a sharp, bevelled tip. They come in two main styles, one has a blade with bevelled edges and the other has a blade with a rectangular cross-section. The sharp tip is prone to damage when abused, such as being used as a levering tool, and can have a highly characteristic profile.

work piece an object that is in the process of being cut, shaped or otherwise being worked on to produce a final product or component.

wrecking bar another term for a *case opener*, crowbar, *pry bar*, and so on, type tool.

wrench although this term can be applied to a variety of tools having fixed or adjustable jaws that are used for gripping, turning, or twisting objects, in this book it is primarily used for hand-held tools designed to grip pipes and pipe fittings. This type of tool is known as a *pipe wrench*. In use, the serrated jaws self-tighten on the object being gripped. As well as the intended use, this type of *wrench* can be used to grip various objects including *padlocks* to force entry. Marks left by a *pipe wrench* would appear as a series of parallel lines on both sides of the gripped item. A *pipe wrench* may also be known as a '*Stilson wrench*' or just 'Stilsons' after the original designer. A *monkey wrench* (or gas grips) has smooth jaws and would fit into this category, but is far less common and would tend to leave apparently featureless marks.

zip-seal bag a specialised *grip-seal bag* where a slide is moved across the bag to close the sealing strips, instead of pressing by hand.

Index

Page numbers in *italics* refer to illustrations

The Forensic Examination and Interpretation of Tool Marks, First Edition.
David Baldwin, John Birkett, Owen Facey and Gilleon Rabey.
© 2013 John Wiley & Sons, Ltd. Published 2013 by John Wiley & Sons, Ltd.